Attention deficit hyperactivity disorder (ADHD) is a common behavioral problem that affects approximately 5% of boys and 1% of girls. It is characterized by a short attention span, trouble concentrating, difficulty sitting still, impulsivity, and other symptoms.

Tourette syndrome is also common and is characterized by the presence of muscle tics, vocal noises, attention deficit hyperactivity disorder, obsessive-compulsive behaviors, learning disorders and conduct problems. Children with ADHD often develop symptoms of Tourette syndrome as they get older.

"Ryan was active when still in the womb. As an infant he did not sleep at night and took no afternoon naps. He did not like to be held, and was irritable, impatient, impulsive, demanding, hyperactive, aggressive, always throwing temper tantrums, and resistant to discipline. Trivial things would send him into a rage. He repeated things over and over, talked too loud, screamed excessively, didn't listen, couldn't take no for an answer, resisted change, punched holes in walls and, on top of all this, seemed totally unaware of the effect his behavior was having on those around him...Life was a roller coaster of good days followed by horrible days, of Dr. Jekyll followed by Mr. Hyde."

Susan Hughes tells of her struggle with understanding Ryan's unusual behaviors, of getting a diagnosis, and of struggling with her own feelings of guilt.

Her message is written in the ultimately understandable language of parent to parent. Written so others need not feel so alone or struggle through so many years of uncertainty.

RYAN
— *A Mother's Story of Her*
Hyperactive/Tourette Syndrome Child

Susan Hughes

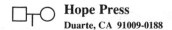 **Hope Press**
Duarte, CA 91009-0188

Disclaimer

This book is designed to provide information in regard to the subject matter covered. It is sold with the understanding that the publisher and author are not engaged in rendering medical, psychiatric, psychological, legal or other professional services to the reader. If such are required, the services of a competent professional in the appropriate field should be sought.

Every effort has been made to make this book as accurate as possible; however, there may be mistakes both typographical and in content. Therefore, this text should be used only as a source of general information and specifics relating to a given individual should be obtained from the services of a professional. Furthermore, this book contains information only up to the printing date.

The purpose of this book is education. Neither the author nor the publisher shall have or accept liability or responsibility to any person or entity with respect to loss or damage or any other problem caused or alleged to be caused directly or indirectly by information contained in this book.

Table of Contents

Foreword

Mothers can be a great source of wisdom. Doctors may listen but they do not always hear what mothers are saying. The story Susan Hughes tells is typical of what thousands of mothers of hyperactive or Tourette syndrome children have endured. The most unusual aspect of her story is that she took the time to write it down — carefully, clearly and eloquently — for the benefit of other mothers who are just beginning a similar journey, or who are reeling from the experience and still don't know what hit them.

Ryan was active when still in the womb. As an infant he did not sleep at night and took no afternoon naps. He did not like to be held, and was irritable, impatient, impulsive, demanding, hyperactive, aggressive, always throwing temper tantrums, and resistant to discipline. Trivial things would send him into a rage. He repeated things over and over, talked too loud, screamed excessively, didn't listen, couldn't take no for an answer, resisted change, punched holes in walls and, on top of all this, seemed totally unaware of the effect his behavior was having on those around him.

By the time school started the first thought was to

wait another year. After being in school, the second thought was to hold him back a year. Although very bright he reversed his words and letters, had horrible handwriting, was disruptive and couldn't concentrate in class. He was hitting and biting other children, pulling and chewing on his clothes, and swearing like a sailor. Although Ritalin brought about a dramatic and miraculous change in his behavior, after several years it seemed to lose its effectiveness. He began sticking out his tongue and developed a "hair out of his eyes tic" and the swearing got worse. Life was a roller coaster of good days followed by horrible days, of Dr. Jekyll followed by Mr. Hyde. Susan first denied there was a problem, then denied he had a neurological disorder, then denied he needed medication. When she finally realized the medication was helping she then felt defensive and guilt-ridden. When her son was finally diagnosed as having Tourette syndrome it was a relief to finally know what the problem was, to have a name for it, and to know his bad behavior was not her fault. While the problems did not all go away, Susan found that the known was much less frightening to deal with than the unknown. The desire to change the unknown to the known for others as well led her to write about her son, Ryan. Her message is written in the ultimately understandable language of parent to parent, so others need not feel so alone or struggle through many years of uncertainty.

David E. Comings, M.D.

Preface

It is my sincere opinion that mothers of hyperactive children who actually survive long enough to see their child graduate from high school should automatically be awarded a Nobel Prize! Surely, any woman who can live on the front lines of that type of combat duty for nearly eighteen years and still have enough energy to tell about it should be considered a modern-day saint!

In addition to the formidable task of living with a child that makes Dennis the Menace look like an angel, these moms often find themselves thrown into a fiery furnace with pediatricians, neurologists, psychologists, psychiatrists, school teachers, principals, tutors, speech therapists and special education directors. They have learned to endure unrelenting humiliation and to smile graciously while being force-fed well meaning, yet unsolicited advice from family, friends, and even strangers. These courageous and misunderstood mothers have learned to swallow criticism by the cupful while saving their tears for those rare, private and quiet times alone.

I have felt for quite sometime that there was a story inside of me that I would like to share. Many times a page has been turned or a chapter inscribed in my mind as I lay in bed late at night wondering what the dawn might bring and if my aching body and spirit would be able to face the light of another morning. Mornings come early to the mother of a hyperactive child, and the days are long. Sometimes too long. But, as I have learned so patiently, with each new day comes new hope and the strength from above to rise to the challenge of caring for that "exceptional" child that God has seen fit to trust in my care. As the old black spiritual laments, "Nobody knows the trouble I've seen."

But this story isn't about trouble. It's about a beautiful and courageous little boy named Ryan whose first nine years have been a triumph over struggles in a world that just doesn't understand.

This book is written especially for all the mothers of hyperactive, Attention Deficit Disorder and Tourette syndrome children. We are sisters through a common bond. We have seen each other in grocery store check out lines and across the table at our local fast-food restaurants and we have known without a doubt that we were related in a very special way. Yes, indeed, we are sisters. God bless us everyone.

Chapter 1

The Perfect Mother Syndrome

She's a woman that most of us women could envy! She's the mother with the adorable blonde-haired, blue eyed, angelic looking toddler who seems to be absolutely perfect! Her child sleeps dutifully through the night when put to bed, and eats only what is offered to her, never asking for more. Her little "angel" smiles at everyone, including strangers, and has a face so adorable that it should be on Gerber baby food jars or at least on magazine covers! Of course, this woman's child is a genius too! At only two and one-half years of age she can work the jumbo twenty-five piece Big Bird puzzles in record time, says please and thank you without being reminded and has been potty-trained for months!

It's hard to believe that I was that woman! I had it all — a wonderful, adoring husband and a beautiful, perfect little girl named Julie. I was feeling happy and wonderfully smug with my parenting role. Nothing to it, I thought. I had read all of the latest parenting books (even the one by Dr. Spock), and obviously I had done all the right things. Our daughter was a joy and a delight and it was all due to my being such a terrific mother! Or so I thought.

1

I was on top of the world. I was thinner than I had been in years, and I was perfectly happy to be a "stay-at-home" mom. McDonalds, Sesame Street and story hour at the library were the highlights in my life now and I was beginning to think seriously about having another child. After all, we enjoyed Julie so much that we easily convinced ourselves that it wouldn't be fair to her to be raised as a "spoiled" only child. It seemed there were so many reasons to have another child and not many reasons not to.

It was with a great deal of joy that we welcomed news of my second pregnancy. Our hopes were for a boy so that we could have the "perfect" American family — one of each, a boy and a girl. But this child was not to be. I suffered a miscarriage early in the third month of pregnancy, and to this day, I think of that little baby and wonder about the child that we never had a chance to know.

It was Thanksgiving time when I learned again that I was expecting. It was an especially happy time of year and Jim and I were anxiously awaiting the Christmas holidays when we were planning to take Julie on a plane to California to see her grandmother and the rest of my family. The weather was lovely and we enjoyed a wonderful Christmas day together with the family, but by the time evening had passed, my happiness had turned to worry and fear.

I had begun to have abdominal cramps and pain much the same as I had experienced with the miscarriage a few months earlier. Also, I had begun to hemorrhage. By the next evening, I was being treated at the hospital for what the emergency room doctor believed to be a tubal pregnancy. I was given a paper to sign for permis-

2

sion to terminate the pregnancy and my husband Jim was asked to do the same. A gynecologist was called in to perform the surgery, but before continuing, he decided to perform a diagnostic procedure called a culdoscopy that hopefully would help to finalize the diagnosis. The culdoscopy was a painful procedure done without anesthesia, but as it turned out, enduring the pain was more than worth it. The doctor was able to determine from the testing that I did not have a tubal pregnancy after all and that there was still a 50/50 chance that I could carry the baby to term! An ultrasound performed the following morning confirmed his diagnosis and I returned home to Cincinnati to wait and see what would happen during the next few critical days.

The next few days turned into the next few weeks, then into several months and I was still pregnant! Although the initial problems with my pregnancy seemed to be over, I had not been gaining much weight throughout this period of time, and even in my seventh month of pregnancy was not "showing" much at all. It was around this time that my doctor began to show concern that the baby may not be growing just as it should be, and I then began what was to become a barrage of diagnostic tests. I was asked to collect my urine in gallon jars and take them into the hospital for testing each week. I also had numerous blood tests, ultrasounds and, finally, the dreaded amniocentesis where a long needle was inserted through my abdomen to collect amniotic fluid for further testing.

By the time eight and one-half months of pregnancy had passed by, I was in sheer misery. This little baby had seemed unusually active and had never stopped boxing and kicking since early in the fourth month! It was impossible for me to sleep at night or for me even to be comfortable throughout the day. It seemed that it was constant kicking and poking and pain, both day and night.

Because my first child, Julie, had been delivered by cesarean section (due to cephalopelvic disproportion), this child too was scheduled to be delivered by cesarean section. But the day before the pre-planned delivery date arrived, an amniocentesis revealed that the baby's lungs were not yet mature and the delivery would have to be postponed. We would have to wait yet another week! As badly as I was feeling, I wasn't at all sure that I would make it through another week!

The doctor was still very concerned about the baby's seemingly small size. Based on his measurements and tests, he estimated the baby to be only about three pounds at most. During these final few weeks I was a bundle of nerves, concerned that there was something wrong with the baby that perhaps the doctor wasn't telling me. I was anxious to get the pregnancy over, no matter what the outcome. I was mentally prepared for the worst but still hoping and praying for the best.

A repeat amniocentesis was scheduled for the following week; however, I unexpectedly went into labor a week early. A neonatalogist was summoned to the delivery room to attend the new little infant that was expected to have potentially serious problems.

At 9:20 a.m. on July 23, 1979, Ryan James Hughes was born, perfectly healthy, weighing in at a hefty six pounds, 11 ounces, much to the surprise of the doctors and to the delight of his parents. He was placed immediately into the arms of his proud and beaming father who was seated by my side.

Little did we know that sunny, summer morning that our lives would be changed so dramatically by that kicking, crying little fireball that wiggled in his father's arms.

Chapter 2
Through the First Year

I remember feeling absolutely euphoric during my first few weeks of being a mother of two. Our beautiful daughter, Julie, had obviously never heard of sibling rivalry and she welcomed her little brother into our home with eagerness and eyes of love, which lasted just until he was old enough to crawl!

Ryan was an exceptionally strong little baby and was very alert from early on. His nap times were few and far between and I remember complaining to the pediatrician about the fact that he was not sleeping through the night at five weeks of age as my first child (the angel) had done. He just chuckled and reminded me that most children don't sleep through the night at such a young age and that perhaps we had just been lucky with the first one. Of course, I didn't want to believe that! I reassured myself that the doctor was probably just teasing and I continued to look forward anxiously to the night when I would manage to wake up and find it to be seven o'clock in the morning instead of two o'clock in the morning. (Little did I know that nine years later I would still be waiting!)

Not only did Ryan continue for many months to awaken several times during the night, but he also had difficulty with his sleeping and nap times throughout the day. Any noise at all would startle him and start him on a crying binge that was difficult to stop. I also found that he was very hard to comfort. He would not permit me or anyone to hold him close for any length of time. He preferred to be held facing away from me, and the more I moved around while holding him, the more he liked it.

I began to notice that different sleeping habits were not the only thing that distinguished Ryan from his sister. Ryan was a very demanding baby. He wanted his food NOW and he would erupt into a crying rage just hearing me open the refrigerator door to get his bottle. It was difficult for me to bring his milk or baby food to even a lukewarm temperature because of his fits of rage. I soon learned to anticipate his little hunger bell and I did my very best to be prepared. Quieting him down was no easy task since he didn't like to cuddle or be rocked. Ryan, as we soon discovered, was allergic to milk but he thrived on soy bean formula and gained weight quickly.

My first year of being the parent of two shot a few arrows of doubt into my puffed-up pride of being the "perfect" mother. By the time Ryan was walking at the age of 12 months, I knew that my halo was already tarnished in spots, but all in all, we were just very thankful to have this healthy, beautiful baby boy in our family.

Chapter 3

The Terribly
Terrible Twos

The terrible twos came early. Almost a year early. When Ryan learned to walk it was the end of our peace of mind! Sibling rivalry reared it's ugly head with a vengeance the day that Ryan first walked on his own steam into his sister's private room. He seemed to sense the feeling of electricity that was created each time he crossed that threshold and it drew him back like a magnet each time he was pulled away!

To say that he was VERY ACTIVE would be an understatement. Like most two year olds, he was into, under, and on top of everything. He was like a little elf with jet engines propelling his legs! He was constantly climbing, jumping or diving head first over the top of something or someone.

By the time he reached eighteen months of age, we had put up those ugly accordion gates in every room in our house in an effort to slow him down. It did no good. The very first day the gates were installed, he learned to dive over the top of them with little effort and he continued on his merry way to unroll the toilet tissue or empty all the drawers in the bedroom dressers. His crib was retired to the garage shortly after his first birthday because he would constantly "dive bomb" over the top of the rails, causing much distress to his tired old mom and dad.

It was very confusing to us around this time that Ryan had such a high pain tolerance. His various escapades often brought many bumps, bruises, scrapes, etc., but he never showed a reaction to injuries. I remember on one occasion that he touched the burner on the electric stove and actually scorched the skin on his finger, yet he didn't cry at all. Many times we would discover minor injuries during his evening bath and we hadn't even been aware that he had hurt himself. He often took some serious falls in his climbing escapades but he would seldom complain or cry.

With my husband, Jim, being a teacher and me being a "stay-at-home" mother, finances were tight in our household during Ryan's early years. Extra money was a pipe dream for us and we lived, as most teachers' families do, from paycheck to paycheck. We had a rather large backyard in our suburban Cincinnati home, but Ryan always preferred the neighbor's yard, and their pool. We knew that for safety's sake we needed to fence in our backyard. We somehow managed to get a loan at our school credit union for a chain link fence to surround our yard, believing that it would provide us some peace of mind while Ryan was playing outdoors.

In order to save money, we put the fence up ourselves. Jim and his brother, Barry, dug each post hole by hand and after several weekends of backbreaking work, our huge backyard was snugly enclosed. How wonderful it was going to be, we thought, to just open the back door and let our little eighteen month old whirlwind out to play in his sandbox without having to worry about his safety! But before the shovels and tools were put away, Ryan had dragged his tricycle over to the fence to investigate. In less than a minute, he had scaled to the top of the four-foot-high fence and, barefooted, had dived head first to the other side. Without even stopping to look back he took off running one hundred miles per hour straight to the next-door neighbor's house with the pool! How stupid we were to think that nearly one thousand dollars worth of galvanized metal would slow down our speeding little bullet!

Ryan continued to be not only fast and active, but also very demanding and aggressive. His high chair became a launching pad for flying food. He would throw everything, including his silverware and plate. We finally learned that securing him in his high chair with a wide, leather man's belt was the safest way of slowing him down for meals. But he was like Houdini when it came to escaping and even our most clever plans were unraveled by his genius and determination.

Hitting, kicking, throwing and biting were becoming more frequent. Even though this child was wearing us both out and putting prematurely gray hairs on our spinning heads, Jim and I tried to assure ourselves that he was just "all boy," that he was strong-willed and that he needed lots of love and discipline.

I was beginning to realize that my self-imposed halo had a definite dent in it, and by this time, it was sitting crooked atop my dizzy head! I began to earnestly scout the local book stores each week for any new "parenting" books.

Chapter 4

Spare the Rod?

Ryan's third birthday party had a "Dukes of Hazzard" motif and his own little engine was every bit as fast and as powerful as the bright orange General Lee. His physical agility was becoming even more pronounced and he used his athletic abilities to conquer every tangible item that crossed his path.

He was an adorable little boy with bright blue eyes and beautiful blonde hair that formed a frame around his pudgy and usually dirty little face. He seemed to be a Dennis the Menace clone not only in appearance, but in his actions too. He was always getting into some kind of trouble.

Just when most children his age were outgrowing the "terrible twos" behavior, Ryan was not. In fact, he seemed to be regressing instead of maturing. His emotions during this time were very volatile and extreme. He would throw, bite or hit on impulse. After playing happily with a toy or with his blocks for a period of time, he would suddenly start into a rage and throw his toys at the television, furniture or at whatever person happened to be in the room at the time.

This would happen for seemingly no apparent reason. He seemed to have an extremely low frustration level with everything and everyone. Temper tantrums were commonplace and they were becoming even more and more frequent, especially in public.

Jim and I both subscribe to Dr. James Dobson's expressed views on Christian parenting and we firmly believed that in certain circumstances children could benefit from a sound spanking on the posterior, especially in instances of willful disobedience. This had worked very effectively with our daughter, Julie, and seldom had we felt it necessary to use corporal punishment during her seven years. Yet spanking Ryan seemed to be like adding gasoline to a fire. Not only was he not remorseful after the punishment, he would be intent on repeating the same misbehavior that initiated the spanking! It became obvious that no matter what we tried as a method of discipline, nothing seemed to work effectively. He did not appear to care or to be affected by whatever punishment we administered.

Our lives were becoming more and more rattled as the months wore on. Ryan seemed to be very excitable and irritable at times. Aggression was becoming more apparent and he would brag on the way home from church about how he knocked down those "babies" at Sunday school. He was beginning to show a frightening disregard for the safety and feelings of others, not only strangers, but his family as well.

Occasionally a friend or family member would ask me if I thought Ryan was hyperactive. I was always quick to assure them that he was not. After all, I reasoned, his dad came from a large family of boys and Ryan was just very active, but certainly not hyper. His grandparents (Jim's mother and father) were very close to Ryan and adored him, no matter how much mischief he caused, and they were quick to defend my point of view. Their grandson, they were quite sure, was just "all boy" and he would certainly grow out of it! By the time Ryan was three and one-half years old, Jim and I were beginning to have serious doubts.

Chapter 5
Mother's Day

I will never forget Mother's Day 1983. After making it through an unusually hectic morning, we were finally on our way to church, running our usual ten minutes late. Julie looked beautiful in her green and white gingham dress and Ryan was dapper in his oxford cloth shirt and his burgundy striped tie that was "just like daddy's."

I had managed to make myself somewhat presentable that morning after refereeing a series of fights between the angelic looking duo and had been successful in camouflaging the milk stains on my nylons and the grape jelly on my navy suit.

I was eagerly awaiting my spiritual "shot in the arm" that our Sunday services so often provided. I knew that our minister would have a special Mother's Day message that morning and I was anxious to bask in the glory of being honored just for being a Mother. After all, everything is perfect on Mother's Day, I naively thought to myself. But something happened during that twenty minute ride to church that quickly snapped me back to reality. Ryan began demanding, in a very loud voice, that he wanted to go to Papaw's house. He insisted that

17

he didn't want to go see these "dumb" babies at Sunday School, as he called them. His demands became more deafening as the miles went by. He began kicking, fighting and tearing at his car seat. Nothing we could say or do would appease him. His beautiful little face was red with rage and perspiration soaked his blonde hair.

He ripped at his shirt and tie and he swung wildly at his sister, who was strapped into the back seat next to him. Nothing we tried would comfort him, not even promises of seeing Papaw right after church, going to McDonald's for a hamburger, or having an ice cream sundae.

By the time we arrived at church that morning, Jim and I were in a state of despair. The Sunday school teacher assured us that he would be fine after we left and we walked on ahead to the sanctuary with Ryan's screams still ringing in our ears.

As the Sunday service began, the Pastor began honoring the "special" mothers who were present that morning. One by one they were asked to stand and receive a yellow rose and a round of applause from the congregation. First, the oldest mother in the congregation, then the youngest, then the one with the most children. I kept waiting for them to call for the mother with the hyperactive three year old. I needed that rose! I needed that round of applause for what I had been through not only that morning, but every morning!

But there was no rose for me that day, and no special recognition. What's so great about being the "youngest" mother, I bemoaned to myself? Doesn't anybody know what *I* put up with every day? Where's MY rose? Self-pity was beginning to eat away at my heart and jealousy of women that I didn't even know was taking hold.

I felt ashamed of myself for being so petty. I began to think of all of the mothers who were suffering as much or even more than I was suffering. I began to think of the mothers whose children were missing or kidnapped and those whose children had been killed in accidents. Also those mothers whose children had died from illnesses or whose children were severely mentally or physically disabled. I soon began to realize that the hurt and pity that I was feeling inside for myself was being felt by other mothers, too, in various types of difficult situations. I was not alone.

Before the Mother's Day service concluded that morning, I was reminded through the hymns of praise of my many blessings. Yes, despite our many difficulties, Jim and I were truly blessed, and a tired but very grateful mother tucked two beautiful children into bed that night.

Chapter 6
Why?

By the time our little son had reached three and one-half years of age, our life as a happy family had begun to crumble before our eyes. We were becoming very much aware that other three year old boys were not quite the same as ours. The Dennis the Menace mischief that we had laughed about when he was two was not quite so funny any more. The blunt truth was that we were going crazy with our child's erratic behavior and we didn't quite know what to do.

Ryan was still hitting, kicking, and biting and he seemed to have practically no impulse control. He still couldn't sit down at meal times, even for a short period of time. He was constantly up and down and would even jump on top of the dinner table while we were eating. No matter how much we spanked, scolded or punished, it didn't seem to deter his impulsive misbehavior. He would throw food or his glass of juice or milk — sometimes right at our faces or sometimes across the room. Believe me, it was very difficult to pick that little boy up from the dinner table, remove him to another room for a harsh spanking and reprimand him only to have him repeat the infraction, not only once but several more

21

times. We tried removing him from the table all together, but he became wild and destructive. We used
various methods of discipline, including standing in the
corner, time outs, taking away privileges, spankings, and
yet nothing seemed to have an effect on Ryan's behavior.

Ryan had begun to have "babbling" spells where he
would repeat certain words over and over. During these
times he seemed to be in another world, totally oblivious
to what he was doing or what was going on around him.
He would talk incessantly, always in an extremely loud
voice, and he would badger us with his insistencies, even
after he had been acknowledged or answered.

He would have episodes when he would begin to
scream or yell incessantly, many times while we were
riding in the car. There were countless instances when
we would have to pull completely off the road because
of the overwhelming distraction of trying to drive with
him screaming and flailing his body in his car seat,
fighting the safety belts that were holding him down.

As the weeks wore on, Ryan's behavior became
increasingly more anti-social. He would lash out at
strangers on impulse. Or he would spontaneously spit on
people as they passed by. On one occasion I recall a
friendly waitress speaking to Ryan and making a comment to us about what a cute little boy he was. Ryan
responded by yelling at her in a loud voice, "Shut up you
big dummy," and then he started to laugh and began his
"babbling," as we called it.

He was totally unpredictable and we had no idea
when he would let out a blood-curdling scream in the
middle of a store or restaurant. With Jim and I being
somewhat quiet and reserved, the humiliation of having

an uncontrollable child became too much to bear and we began to stay at home whenever possible.

I will never forget the many times that we dragged a screaming child into a public restroom and spanked him until we knew it was not possible to spank him anymore without causing him serious harm. But it didn't seem to matter. This tiny little three year old had a pain tolerance that was unbelievable! Nothing that we could do to him, or say to him, had any impact.

Our nerves were frayed. I emphasize "our" nerves, because Jim and I were equally committed and involved with Ryan throughout this difficult time. Although we were both mature and reasonably intelligent adults, we had dipped into the bottom of our well of intellectual resources for an answer and we were coming up dry and empty.

There was one particular week in May 1983 that I will never forget. A series of events helped to reinforce in our minds what we had tried for so long to deny. Within the span of seven days Ryan managed to:

1. Set off the fire alarm at church.
2. Tried to pull a gun out of a policeman's holster who was waiting in a line in front of us.
3. Threw a toy at his sister's face, causing her to have seven stitches just below the eye.
4. Broke his grandfather's garage window by hurling a tennis ball at it.
5. Shattered a plateglass mirror in a department store while strapped in his stroller.

All of these things were done while his father and I were standing right next to him! He was as quick as lightning and even the two of us together could not anticipate fast enough, or act quickly enough, to stop his impulsive actions. All of these incidents in the course of a week, combined with the other behaviors we were dealing with at home, forced us to realize that we needed HELP!

Our little son had also become unable to listen or to communicate in a normal manner. And throughout all of these ordeals, he seemed to be totally unaware of the fact that he was doing anything wrong. He did not appear to be cognitive in the least, despite any form of discipline, that he was driving everyone crazy. He had absolutely no awareness of the magnitude of the impact of his behavior on his family or others.

At the point of helplessness and despair we phoned our pediatrician for a consultation appointment. For the first time in our lives, we were going to bare our souls to another person regarding our seemingly poor parenting skills. After all, it must be our fault, we reasoned. Why else would this beautiful little child have such aberrant behavior?

"Why? Why?" I asked myself over and over. I asked God over and over. "What can we do to help him Lord," I prayed. "Please give us the answer. What are we going to do? How can we help him," I questioned.

With a pound of helplessness and an ounce of hope, we drove to the doctor's office wondering if our lives would ever be normal again.

Chapter 7
Minimal Brain What?

The pediatrician who had been treating Ryan was a well-respected physician in Cincinnati, Ohio. We had been referred to him by an acquaintance who was a nurse in the pediatric surgery department of Children's Hospital in Cincinnati. On our first visit to his office I was further reassured of his qualifications by reading in a local magazine article that he had been named one of the top three pediatricians in the city in a vote taken by his fellow associates.

Although we had seen this doctor for all of the usual childhood complaints (including "thousands" of ear infections), as Jim and I sat in his office for our consultation appointment, I felt nervous and unsure of the wisdom in our being there. Pangs of doubt jabbed at my mind and I wondered if he would smirk or laugh when we told him that we were unable to control our small three year old son. Even admitting that to myself seemed ridiculous. Surely two reasonably intelligent, mature adults, such as Jim and I could control a child of only thirty pounds. "What's wrong with you Susan, are you crazy, or just stupid," I admonished myself.

As I began to mentally berate and punish myself for

being such a horrible parent, I slowly became aware of the reasons we had made the appointment in the first place. Our home life had become miserable! We were not able to do any of the normal things that families do. Ryan's behavior had become so horrible in public that we had been forced to stay at home with him for weeks. It was impossible to even go to McDonald's for a hamburger without a major catastrophe. And, to make matters worse, staying home for meals was no better. Ryan would not (or could not) sit down and be still long enough to eat, whether alone or with the three of us. He would jump up on top of the table, throw his food, scream, yell, cry, badger, kick, knock things off the table, try to turn the table over, try to tip his chair over backwards, spill his drink, and spit his food.

Bedtime was also difficult because he would awaken many times through the night crying or screaming. He would thrash his bed covers all over during the night and he never seemed able to rest peacefully. In the mornings he would awaken early (five thirty-ish) and begin the day with loud demands for breakfast, but would never seem to be able to wait long enough for me to get the food to him. His days were filled with chaotic, frenetic activity, always running, racing, climbing, jumping and throwing. He was unable to take no for an answer without becoming violent. And the babbling spells had become more and more frequent. There was no doubt about it. We had to talk to someone. We just couldn't continue on like this.

The pediatrician talked with Jim and me for over an hour and a half. He questioned us at length about Ryan's behavior and our methods of discipline. He took lots of notes and from his line of questioning, I could sense that he was genuinely concerned about our situation. Because Ryan had not yet started school, the doctor asked if perhaps Ryan's Sunday school teacher would fill out a questionnaire that would describe his behavior in a group situation. He also scheduled us to come back in a few days in order that he could give Ryan a complete physical examination and check for "soft" neurological signs.

After reviewing the Sunday school teacher's report (which noted much aggression with the other children and excessive motor activity), the doctor gave Ryan a thorough check up from head to toe. During the visit Ryan began one of his "spells" and he began to repeat "Mom-mee, Mom-mee, Mom-mee," over and over again, becoming louder each time. I was holding him on my lap at the time and all attempts I made to quiet him were to no avail. He began to paw at me like a dog or a kitten and he would not stop. He started to pull at my clothing as if I were a tree and he was trying to pull himself up the bark. Nothing that I could say or do seemed to matter. This went on for several minutes and eventually it began to subside with Ryan slowly beginning to assume a degree of self control. As the doctor was preparing to leave the examining room, I stopped him, asking about the "soft" neurological signs that he had mentioned he would be checking for. The doctor answered me by saying emphatically, "Believe me Mrs. Hughes, your son has LOUD neurological signs."

As I followed him into his office to hear the verdict of his exam, I was thoroughly confused about the comment, but was glad that he was able to see for himself some of the behavior that we were experiencing at home.

When I had settled myself and Ryan into the small chair in the doctor's private office, he began by saying that it appeared that Ryan had a neurological disorder known as Minimal Brain Dysfunction. Anything that he said for the next few sentences became a blur to me. I could faintly hear his voice speaking, as if he were far away, but the only thing that registered in my mind were the words: minimal brain dysfunction.

"Wait a minute," I thought to myself. This doctor is telling me that there is something wrong with my child's brain! Just who in the world does he think he is," I wondered. "He must be out of his mind! Just because Ryan has a behavior problem doesn't mean there's something wrong with his brain," I protested silently.

My defenses went up immediately, and as I focused back onto the doctor's voice, I heard him saying that medication was often very effective in treating children with this disorder. He was suggesting a trial use of a stimulant medication, called Ritalin, and he was waiting for me to respond.

I managed to get control of my racing mind and politely informed the doctor that Jim and I would prefer *not* to medicate our three year old child. I assured him that we would continue to try harder to cope with his behavior and to make an effort to be more consistent with our discipline at home. Also, I explained to him that I had heard something about the Feingold diet for hyperactive children and I suggested to him that if we would better police the food colorings, additives and sugars in Ryan's diet perhaps things may possibly improve. Although the doctor assured me that there was absolutely no scientific evidence that diet was directly related to hyperactivity, and that I could spend three hours in the largest supermarket in town and find only a few items without any of those ingredients that a three year old would eat, he gave in to my persistence of giving the diet another try.

Before we left his office the doctor again offered his advice. "Mrs. Hughes," he began sympathetically, "I have mothers who come into my office and literally beg me to give them medication because they suspect their child is hyperactive. Yet, when I do an examination and workup, I find that their children are perfectly normal. But your son NEEDS medication, and to be perfectly honest, I don't understand why you are not at least willing to give it a try. Here is a pamphlet on Minimal Brain Dysfunction. Please call me when you are ready."

I lasted less than a week. Each day was worse than the day before. Despite desperate attempts at a very consistent discipline program, and another try at eliminating food coloring and additives, things were no better. On the day that I called the doctor back, I had stood Ryan in the corner fifteen times before twelve noon. I had resolved to be consistent in my discipline and also in the rewards that were planned for good behavior. But there was no good behavior to reward that morning and trying to get him to stand in the corner for five minutes for fifteen different times was more than I could handle! There had also been several spankings in between for infractions such as picking up the kitchen stool and throwing it at me, kicking his sister in the stomach, and putting a hole in the wall of his bedroom. I had also tried to isolate him in his room, but he had become violent and I was afraid that he would hurt himself or even Julie or me.

The pediatrician suggested that we try two and one-half milligrams of Ritalin when Ryan first got up the next morning. I nearly choked from the lump in my throat when I gave my little boy that half-piece of the round yellow pill for the first time. He swallowed it with ease, and I bent over and kissed his head. "I love you R.J.," I said, somehow believing that my loving him would justify my failure as a mother that was causing him to take medication. You see, I still felt very much to blame for his behavior, despite the doctor's explanation of a neurological disorder.

I was to report back to the doctor later in the afternoon for a progress report. But nothing much had changed. After one day on medication, there was no significant change. The doctor said to increase the medication to a whole tablet the next morning, which would be five milligrams. Again, as he swallowed the tiny pill, I kissed his head and said, "I love you Ryan." But this morning, surprisingly enough to me, seemed to go a little more smoothly than usual. In fact, it was great! Ryan played with his Legos, watched Sesame Street and even ate an early lunch with no major problems. But soon after the noon hour, things were back to normal again and Ryan was being his "usual" self.

Things went on this way for the next few days. The mornings were great, but the afternoons were terrible. When checking in with the doctor at the end of the week, he suggested that we try giving Ryan a half of a five milligram tablet around noon. That seemed to help a bit, but by dinner time things had deteriorated quite a bit. Yet, we were totally amazed at the child who lived with us in the mornings from eight to twelve. He was perfectly normal! He talked, he played, he ate and he behaved in a perfectly normal manner. But the child who lived in that same body from twelve noon until bedtime was a wild child. When the doctor recommended, over a period of time, increasing the noon dosage to five milligrams, and adding a third dose at four in the afternoon, we did not question.

The difference in Ryan's behavior when he was on medication was the difference between night and day. It was absolutely unbelievable! It was awesome to think that a tiny yellow pill could make life worth living again. We had our son back! A beautiful, fun-loving, active but normal little boy lived with us now and he was a joy, at least for most of the day

It seemed that there was a slight problem with the medication wearing off. The pills were supposed to last four hours, but they only lasted three to three and one-half hours, at most; yet he could only take the pills no sooner than every four hours. Then after taking a pill, it would sometimes take twenty minutes before it would start to work its magical spell. So there were often periods of sometimes an hour or so when Ryan was not under full control of the medication. These times were extremely noticeable. We never needed a watch to know when it was time for the next dose. Ryan's behavior was the indicator. We could tell exactly by his actions and the tone of his voice when it was time for the next pill.

It was a short time later that I spotted a small article in an issue of *Better Homes & Gardens* magazine outlining the correlation of children using the drug Ritalin with the onset of a neurological disorder known as Tourette syndrome. I made a mental note to ask the pediatrician about it as one of the symptoms mentioned was rapid eyeblinking, which Ryan had done briefly during the first few days he had begun taking Ritalin.

When I queried the doctor about the article months later, he was quick to assure me that Tourette syndrome would develop only in children who were already pre-disposed to the condition and not to worry about Ritalin causing any problems. I remember him saying in a very matter-of-fact tone, "Mrs. Hughes, let me assure you that *Better Homes & Gardens* has never been an authority on pediatric neurology and you really shouldn't worry about everything you read."

I concluded that he was probably right. I certainly didn't need to borrow trouble by worrying about some disorder that I'd never even heard of before. I was so very relieved that Ryan had shown such improvement with the medication. Jim and I were both elated that most days were going really well and we were thrilled that medical science was able to offer some quality to our family life!

Chapter 8
Ritalin and Ryan

It had been several months since Ryan had begun taking Ritalin and although our family life had become more normal, due to the dramatic transformation in Ryan's behavior, I was suffering from a terminal case of the "guilts." I just couldn't escape the nagging little voice that seemed to whisper, "Shame on you Susan. . . what kind of a mother are you to drug your child? It's going to damage his liver, or worse yet, he's going to become a druggee — a drug addict. First Ritalin and then the big H — heroine. And it's going to be your fault for being such a rotten mother!!!!"Of course,in my mind I knew better, but the little pangs of doubt seemed to be getting stronger and stronger.

One day my friend called to tell me that she had listened to Dr. James Dobson's radio program, called "Focus on the Family," that morning and that the subject had been on hyperactivity. She suggested that I send for a copy of the tape. I decided to phone in my order instead of writing, and in just a few short days I received the audio tape in the mail.

Hearing that message on tape was just what I needed! Dr. Dobson was describing Ryan exactly! He even talked of the guilt that I was feeling and it seemed at the time that his comments were aimed directly at me. His views on the effective use of medications for hyperactive children were discussed, and later, when reading Dr. Dobson's book, *The Strong Willed Child*, I sensed a tremendous wave of relief when I realized, for the first time, that someone else actually understood what I was going through! When reading the chapter entitled, "The Problem with Hyperactivity" (Or Jiggle, Jump, Climb and Roll on the Floor), it seemed as if Dr. Dobson was describing Ryan perfectly when he defined hyperactivity:

"Hyperactivity, (also called hyperkinesis, minimal brain dysfunction, impulse disorder, and at least thirty other terms) is defined as excessive and *uncontrollable* movement. It usually involves distractibility, restlessness, and a short attention span. I italicized the word uncontrollable because the severely affected child is absolutely incapable of sitting quietly in a chair or slowing down his level of activity. He is propelled from within by forces he can neither explain nor ameliorate."

In answering the question, "How Early Can the Problem be Identified," Dr. Dobson continued by saying:

"The severely hyperactive child can be recognized during early toddlerhood. In fact, he can't be ignored. By the time he is thirty months of age he may have exhausted his mother, irritated his siblings, and caused the grandparents to retire from babysitting duties. No family mem-

34

ber is 'uninvolved' with his problem. Instead of growing out of it, as the physician may promise, he continues to attack his world with the objective of disassembling it"

Dr. Dobson described my sentiments with accuracy when answering the query, "How Do Parents React?":

"The mother of a hyperactive child typically experiences a distressing tug of war in her mind. On the one side, she understands her child's problem and feels a deep empathy and love for her little fellow. There is nothing that she wouldn't do to help him. But on the other side, she resents the chaos he has brought into her life. Speedy Gonzales spills his milk and breaks vases and teeters on the brink of disaster throughout the day. He embarrasses his mother in public and shows little appreciation for the sacrifices she is making on his behalf. By the time bedtime arrives, she often feels as if she has spent the entire day in a foxhole.

What happens, then, when genuine love and strong resentment collide in the mind of a mother or father? The inevitable result is parental guilt in sizeable proportions — guilt that is terribly destructive to a woman's peace of mind and even to her health."

In discussing the issue of medications in the treatment of hyperactive children, Dr. Dobson offered this counsel:

"There are dozens of medications which have been shown to be effective in calming the hyperactive child. Since every child's chemistry is unique, it may be necessary for a physician to 'fish' for the right substance and dosage. Let me stress that I am opposed to the administration of such drugs to children who do not require them. In some instances these substances have been given indiscriminately to children simply because their parents or teachers preferred them sedated, which is inexcusable. Every medication has a side effect (even aspirin) and should be administered only after careful evaluation and study. However, if your child displays the symptoms I have described in the preceding section and has been evaluated by a neurologist or other knowledgeable physician, you should not hesitate to accept his prescription of medication. Some dramatic behavioral changes can occur when the proper substance is identified for a particular child."

After reading Dr. Dobson's book, *The Strong Willed Child*, I felt as if my ankles had been cut free from a ball and chain. Here was a well-known author, psychologist, former professor of pediatrics at the University of Southern California School of Medicine, and a prominent Christian leader who I had admired for years actually discussing the problem of hyperactivity in his book and recommending, in instances such as ours, that medication would be appropriate.

Dr. Dobson's expressed views were invaluable to me at that period in my life. Although his opinion echoed that of Ryan's pediatrician and what I already knew in my heart to be true, it was the confirmation that I needed at the time.

Ryan had begun preschool that September and I was thoroughly enjoying the quiet and peaceful three mornings a week that he was away. Things were going fairly well with the medication; however, we could always tell when it was time for the next dose. His tone and behavior would change that dramatically. The pre-school teacher reported no serious problems, but she commented that he seemed to be very distractible and that he needed quite a bit of individual supervision.

Ryan had started to express an interest in learning the letters of the alphabet and he was already able to spell a few words including his name. One evening while out shopping we stopped for a red light in front of a large department store named ZAYRES. All of a sudden Ryan began to yell, "There's my name mommy, there's my name!" I looked all around but couldn't find his name on anything. He became more excited and persisted, "There it is mommy, there's my name." I turned to the back seat and saw that his little finger was pointing to the large neon sign that said ZAYRES. "That's not your name Ryan," I mumbled. "Yes, it is mommy," he insisted. "Look, it says R Y A N on it." It took me a few minutes and then I finally saw what Ryan had readily seen from first glance. He was reading the first four letters of the word backwards, and in his mind, he was seeing the Z as an N. <u>Z A Y R</u> E S

As I drove home I thought of the booklet that the pediatrican had given me on Minimal Brain Dysfunction and how it had described associated learning disabilities that were possible with the disorder, such as dyslexia. I wondered if this was how dyslexia might begin. Ryan was not very adept at printing letters yet, but when he did write, most of his letters were either backwards or upside down (see figures insert). Thinking of this brought another thought to my mind. Ryan often reversed words in a sentence or he would say the opposite of what he actually meant to say. For example, he would declare, "I want to hold you mommy," meaning of course that he wanted me to hold him. Also, he would say that he wanted to come out when he really meant that he wanted to come in. I concluded that it was too early to be concerned. He would probably grow out of these tendencies before time for him to start school.

Ryan continued to have an endless supply of energy. Although medication gave us many normal hours through the day, we still experienced enough of the bad hours to remember what it was like B.R. (Before Ritalin). Ryan seemed to do best when everything followed a routine. Wavering from his established pattern would usually set him off in a rage. I remember well how difficult it was for him to switch from wearing short-sleeved shirts to long-sleeved shirts when the chilly winter days came. And if we dared to drive a different way to Papaw's house or to the grocery store it could start a major conflict that would take hours to resolve.

That winter proved to be an especially trying time for our family. In January I entered the hospital for a total hysterectomy and although the doctor recommended a six week recovery, he obviously didn't realize that hyperactive children do not allow their mothers to be sick at all, let alone have a recuperation time! I resumed my motherly role almost immediately, complete with hot flashes and, in practically no time, I was once again driving the car pool to preschool and baking cookies for

Girl Scouts!

It was soon after my return home from the hospital that Jim's father became seriously ill. Less than six weeks later he died from a painful struggle with lung cancer. Papaw Hughes had been Ryan's best friend. It was Papaw who could comfort Ryan at times when no one else could and the feelings of love shared between the two of them were mutual. Papaw Hughes loved all of his grandchildren, but he seemed to have a special way with this unique little grandson of his. When the rest of us were at our wits end with Ryan's antics, it was always Papaw who would admonish us and say, "Aw, leave him alone, he'll be okay."

Papaw's love for Ryan was blind. He saw only the positives and he talked often about how smart Ryan was. It was Papaw who first put a baseball bat in Ryan's hand at the age of two and it was Papaw who, in ill health, continued to pitch ball after ball to the persistent little fellow waiting patiently in the grassy backyard.

At only four years of age, Ryan lost an important part of his life. It took him months to verbalize his feelings about losing his grandfather. I am still not sure that he really understands, but he does remember and he talks about the fun they had together. Those memories of times with Papaw are something he can keep forever.

One of the things that always amazed us (and Papaw Hughes) about Ryan was his natural ability to handle a baseball. He had always been very adept at catching, batting and, especially, throwing a ball. One day that spring, I noticed in the local paper that Little League sign ups were starting soon. When I read further, I saw that the minimum starting age was five years old.

It was late March by then and Ryan would not be five for over four months yet.

Jim and I decided that we would approach the league managers and ask if they would consider giving Ryan an opportunity to at least try, even though he was only four years old. We tried to convince them that he was really a good little ball player and that he would probably be able to handle the challenge of playing on a team just fine. I'm not quite sure when they quit shaking their heads no and finally said yes, but eventually we persuaded the league officials to take our registration money and consent to try Ryan out on a team. We agreed that if he was unable to keep up with the other players, we would pull him out immediately and wait until the following year.

The whole baseball community in our small rural town knew that the best coach in the league was a woman coach named Sherry. Sherry had been coaching for several years and she always had a winning team. She had a reputation of being great with the kids and for really teaching them a lot about the game. We were elated when Sherry called to tell us that Ryan was going to be on HER team! She was quick to remind us that this was a trial only, after all, he was only four years old.

It took only one practice for Sherry to fall in love with Ryan! "I can't believe the arm on that kid, " she said! "I hate it, but I'm going to have to play him in the outfield though, since he's so little. I'm afraid he'll get hurt." Ryan proved himself to be an able batter and only once during the whole season did he have to hit off the T. But there was one minor, little problem. After making a really good solid hit, Ryan would run to third base instead of first! So Sherry started standing behind him at home plate, and when he hit the ball, she would run up the first base line with him!

Ryan's first year of baseball was a tremendous success. He was able to contribute to the team's success with his good throwing arm and batting, and he learned from a very good teacher the fundamentals of the game and an introduction to sportsmanship. The baseball season ended with a party for the boys and shiny gold trophies for all. Ryan's first picture in a baseball uniform at four years of age is one I will treasure always!

The many struggles during the previous year brought home to our minds the importance of having a strong and loving support system from other family members. Trying to take care of Ryan's special needs by ourselves was very hard for Jim and me. Although Mamaw Hughes was more than willing to help, her age and her health prevented her from offering us the kind of physical help that we so desparately needed.

With my hysterectomy I had struggled to regain my physical and emotional health while still trying to care for Julie and coping with Ryan's problems. We realized that it would be better for us to live closer to my family, in order to have more help with Ryan, and we began to make plans to move to California where my mother, sister, and numerous aunts, uncles and cousins were living. We also thought that the change in climate would help with the numerous allergy and sinus problems that Julie and I had been plagued with for so many years. It seemed that one of us was always coughing with bronchitis or asthma and the thought of the sunny California sun seemed like paradise to us. We packed up our small compact car and headed west in June of 1984. Several months earlier, Jim had sent out approximately twenty applications to school districts in various communities that we thought would be nice areas in which to live. After being in California for only a couple of weeks, Jim was offered a teaching position in a beautiful coastal town just fifty miles north of Los Angeles.

We quickly returned to Ohio to load up our furniture, ecstatic that Jim had found a job so quickly. Both of the children were excited about moving to California and of course Ryan became "overly" excited. The moving truck had only been in the driveway less than five minutes when he rode his tricycle up the ramp, promptly fell off, cut his head open and had to go to the doctor's office for stitches!

Although our home in Cincinnati had not yet sold, we mustered up faith that everything would work out for the best. We managed to stuff all of our earthly belongings into that twenty foot, bright yellow Ryder moving truck, and started out on the long, twenty-five hundred mile journey toward our new home.

Chapter 9
Five Years Old Means
... Kindergarten?

Before moving into our new home in Southern California, Jim and I had wrestled with a difficult decision. Should we start Ryan in kindergarten or should we wait another year and give him a chance to mature? His late July birthday meant that he would be a "young" five year old, and combined with his other difficulties, waiting the extra year would have seemed the most logical thing to do. In addition to these considerations, holding your child back from kindergarten had become a real popular trend — it was the "vogue" thing to do in our community in Ohio and it seemed that many of our new California neighbors shared the same philosophy.

But being a creature of instinct (as most mothers are!) I felt that another year at home with good old mom was not necessarily the best thing for Ryan, or for me. Despite all of our difficulties with his behavior, Ryan seemed to be a very bright child! It seemed logical to me that he needed some added motivation and stimulation that I, alone, could not provide. He was not at all receptive to any attempts that I made to read with him or to play with him. It was evident to me that he needed that "something" more that I was not able to give.

It was with much thought and deliberation that we came to the decision to enroll Ryan for half-day morning kindergarten that fall. The elementary school was only a few short blocks from our home and I loved being close enough to walk with both of the children to school each morning. Ryan always walked briskly, kicking the garbage cans on his way, or taking time to jump in every mud puddle he could find.

Ryan's kindergarten teacher was a very nice woman who, as it turned out, was the wife of the minister at the church we had started attending. She was very helpful and sympathetic to Ryan's problems and she offered him as much individual attention as was possible in a class of thirty-three noisy little five year olds.

Things went smoothly the first couple of months of school, no major catastrophes with behavior or school work. Ryan was taking approximately thirty milligrams of Ritalin per day by this time and it seemed to be doing the job. It was just before the Christmas holidays that the teacher began to note an increase in Ryan's activity level and a decrease in his attention span. We began adjusting the medication and I started helping out in the classroom in order that I could see first-hand some of the problems the teacher had mentioned.

It was evident from the very beginning of my visits to the classroom that printing and coloring were very difficult for Ryan. As I walked between the rows of seats, glancing at the other students' papers, I became very much aware that Ryan's work was the sloppiest, although most of the time the answers he gave were correct. There were a lot of letter reversals in his work: i.e., d for b, p for q, saw for was, etc.

Since Ryan had first been diagnosed as having Attention Deficit Disorder (the new name for Minimal Brain Dysfunction), I had scoured the libraries and book stores for literature on the disorder. One of the first things I learned about was the very high percentage of hyperactive children who also experienced learning disabilities in some form or degree of severity. With Jim being a public school teacher, we were aware that special education programs existed for children who needed extra help and we discussed our concerns with Ryan's teacher. She agreed that a formal assessment would be in order and she started the paperwork for testing to begin.

The school psychologist was efficient and swift in administering the psychological tests and getting back to us with the results. Ryan had done remarkably well on most of the tests with his scores ranging from average to high average and even a scatter to the bright range in some areas. In the area of visual memory, however, Ryan's ability far surpassed his performance, showing just enough discrepancy to qualify him for some individualized tutoring for fifteen minutes per day. The psychologist commented that despite his mostly successful test scores, she felt that Ryan was at extremely high risk for learning disabilities and she recommended his placement in the resource "pull out" program for the remainder of the year. In May, Ryan's progress was to be evaluated and the need for future placement would be made at that time.

In the meantime, behavior problems were becoming more evident at school and at home. Despite medication adjustments things were deteriorating. It seemed that the Ritalin was working for only two and one-half to three hours yet we could still only give him a pill every four hours. Ryan also began wetting his pants through the day, not just once, but usually several times. Even though there was a restroom right in the kindergarten classroom, Ryan came home with wet pants almost every day. The same thing was happening at home. Ryan would wet his pants while watching television, while playing with a friend, while eating, or just anytime! It didn't seem to bother him a bit; in fact, most of the time he didn't even seem to notice that he had done it.

It was during these same months that Ryan became more and more aggressive and abusive. His defiance was maddening and Jim and I struggled to make sense of what was happening. Yes the Ritalin was still working — at least part of the time. There were still very definite times during the day that we had a normal child. Yet the "other child" seemed to be with us more and more often.

I think that perhaps the hardest problem we were dealing with was his seeming lack of impulse control. Many times Ryan would dash into the street right in front of an oncoming car, or he would throw something through the wall of his room in anger. And conceivably, the most frightening episode of all was having him open the car door while we were driving down the crowded freeway! He was also hitting and throwing again on impulse and living with him was like walking on eggs. We never knew what was going to set him off or what he was going to do or say next.

When we had first moved to our new city, we had asked several people to recommend a pediatrician. Much to our surprise, they all named the same doctor. We were quite pleased with Ryan's new physician and we were relieved that the transition from the previous doctor to this one had gone smoothly. The new pediatrician showed immediate concern for Ryan's small size. He was not even "on" the standardized growth chart for height or weight and the doctor encouraged us to bring him in every three months for a complete physical and to keep a check on his growth.

We were all very much aware that one of the side effects of using Ritalin was the possible slowing of growth and it was a concern that we all shared. It was during one of our routine check-ups that Ryan's pediatrician recommended that we consult a psychologist to help with some of the behavior problems we were having. In addition, we started using the time-released Ritalin which would hopefully offer more sustained and even control of his behavior throughout the day.

Ryan loved the psychologist! We went for visits on a regular basis until the doctor became familiar with Ryan and our situation in general. Although he offered no real solutions to our difficult problems, I must admit that it helped me just to talk to someone, especially someone who was sympathetic and who seemed to understand what we were going through. The doctor seemed to establish a good rapport with Ryan and, before too long, we had cut our visits down to an "as needed" basis. Our lives seemed to be on a perpetual roller coaster. Some days were good, some days were impossible. Some weeks were bearable, some weeks were suicidal. But we were coping and learning daily the meaning of taking just "one day at a time."

By the time May rolled around and the school year was drawing to a close, more decisions were to be made.

It was the recommendation of the school assessment team that Ryan repeat kindergarten. Although he had done quite well, they felt that due to his problems with fine motor skills and his social immaturity that another year would help in his development, and we agreed.

What Jim and I had anticipated when first enrolling Ryan for kindergarten the previous September had come to pass. Ryan needed an extra year to mature. Yet, we were so very grateful that we had given him the opportunity to try and we were happy with the many successes that he had experienced. But, despite our feelings that Ryan needed some extra time, we were just a bit hesitant to agree to another year of just kindergarten. Was that really what was best? What, if any, were the alternatives? As far as the school was concerned, repeating kindergarten was the only alternative. But something just didn't "feel" right (mother's instinct again!).

After much thought and agonizing in our minds over what to do, Jim and I agreed that we would approach the school administrators with a different idea. Instead of having Ryan attend only a kindergarten class again, would they perhaps be willing to consider having him attend kindergarten in the morning and attending a first-grade class in the afternoon? We proposed a kind of "combination" year that would provide him with those "extra" months he needed before he would be ready to start into a regular first-grade class the following fall.

We were delighted that our suggestion was met with curious interest and openness. After much discussion it was agreed that Ryan would begin a trial year of kindergarten and first grade. His mornings would be an exact repeat of the previous year. Same work, same teacher, same hours, same everything. Except that, hopefully, things would be much easier the second time around and the expected success would afford Ryan with a much needed boost to his self-confidence and self esteem.

Then, instead of going home at eleven-thirty in the morning, Ryan would report to his first- grade classroom where his classmates were lining up to go to lunch. After having lunch and recess as a full-fledged first grader, Ryan would then go back to class with the other students where afternoon activities would consist of library, computer, show and tell, arts & crafts, nutrition, etc. All of the first-grade afternoon activities were to be non-academic, thus creating no academic pressures that Ryan might not be ready to face.

The idea seemed like it would work but only time would tell. School officials cautioned that this would be done on a "trial" basis only and that if the "experiment" did not work out, Ryan would go back to attending kindergarten only. Jim and I were not sure either how things would work out. We only knew that providing Ryan with a situation that offered him an opportunity for success while still providing him a challenge seemed to make more sense than what could possibly be a boring year of repeating only the same kindergarten material and feeling like a failure in the process.

We were anxious to start the new school year, and thanks to Ritalin, the pediatrician, the psychologist and lots of loving support from family members, we made it through those three long months of summer.

Chapter 10
The Transition Year

Ryan was thrilled that he was going to be able to go to first grade *and* kindergarten. His social immaturity allowed him to accept his placement with eagerness and he never once questioned that he was "different" from the other children. And evidently it was no big deal to the other students either. They neither joked nor teased. His fellow kindergarten classmates were impressed that he was allowed to stay in school with the big kids in the afternoon, and his first-grade peers accepted him into their fold one hundred percent.

The first-grade teacher was well experienced and she ruled her class with a firm hand. She was quick to intervene when Ryan's behavior became a challenge and I'm sure that her expertise prevented many potential problems.

It was during this year of school that Ryan began to spit again. In addition to wetting his pants throughout the day he began to spit at people or just spit into the air for no reason at all. It didn't seem to happen in any type of a pattern. Sometimes he would just be sitting, watching TV, and he would look up and start spitting. We also noticed that when he became frustrated or angry he

51

would start spitting, usually several times. Even though he was doing fairly well on his medication, taking no for an answer was still something that he could just not handle and he would often fly into an uncontrollable rage if things were not going his way.

I was taken a back one day that year when I received a disturbing call from the special education teacher at school. It seemed that one of Ryan's drawings had come to her attention and, in her opinion, was of great concern. She indicated that she had shown the drawing to the school psychologist and that it was their joint conclusion that we should consult Ryan's psychologist regarding the drawing because it suggested much anger and hostility.

I was in tears when I hung up the phone. I was totally confused! Ryan's drawings had always been immature, and his difficulty with fine motor skills made coloring difficult, but surely the teacher wouldn't have called if it wasn't something very serious! I was even more confused when I saw the drawing that was causing the teacher so much alarm.

It was a crude drawing of a stick figure, done with a black crayon. The teacher had been concerned because it was done all in black. But I remembered that on the particular day Ryan had scribbled the drawing we had been seated at a local restaurant, waiting for our food, and I gave Ryan a piece of paper to draw on in an effort to keep him quiet. When reaching into my purse, I found I had only a black crayon, which was the reason he used only black!

We did make an appointment with the psychologist and took the drawing in for his opinion. He started to laugh and said, "I don't see any cause for alarm. This drawing is perfectly normal for a hyperactive child! Perhaps if a normal child had drawn this type of picture I would have been a little more concerned, but certainly not for a child with Ryan's disorder!"

Although I felt much better about the drawing episode, we were still troubled by the spitting, the worsening temper tantrums and the impulsivity that was becoming such a problem again. Because of the continuing babbling spells that we described, the pediatrician recommended that Ryan have an electroencephalogram (brain wave test) taken and he scheduled the test to be done at a local hospital.

We were advised before showing up for the EEG to give Ryan his medication as usual. I wondered at the time why he should be given the medication. It seemed to me that the doctor would want to test his brain waves without the effects of the medication, but I dutifully did as I was instructed and gave Ryan his normal morning dose of Ritalin. I was more nervous about the test than Ryan was, but I managed to mask my feelings and was able to convince Ryan that having the EEG was no big deal.

Ryan was thrilled when the hospital technicians gave him a toy puppet to keep. And he was amused when they put "toothpaste" in his hair to hold the electrodes in place on his head. I was surprised when the testing began that he was able to hold so still. I hadn't seen him that still in his entire life!

Shortly after the testing began, it seemed that the technician was having problems of some sort. It appeared that the EEG machine was being temperamental.

The test only lasted about ten or fifteen minutes, but during the whole time she fussed at the machine, even banging on it with her fist on several occasions in attempt to get it to work properly. When she was finally finished she told us that the doctor would have the report back in his office the next day and that I should call him for the results. "Are you sure that machine is working properly?" I asked, confused that what I thought was a delicate procedure could be done on such a rattly old machine. "Oh sure," she said, "everything's fine. I got what I needed."

I left the hospital totally unconvinced that any reading from that machine could be trusted! But more than that, I was worried that perhaps something would be found wrong with Ryan that might indicate something more serious than "just" hyperactivity.

When I called the doctor's office the next afternoon to learn the results, his nurse replied, "The EEG came back essentially normal Mrs. Hughes. Nothing to worry about." As I hung up the phone a wave of emotion rippled through me. I felt relief — relief that there was no epilepsy or seizure disorder, yet I felt confused as I wondered again about the validity of the results on what seemed to be an unreliable piece of equipment.

I also felt pangs of discouragement. If Ryan did not have any type of a seizure disorder, why was he having those babbling spells? And why was he spitting at people and things for no reason? And why wasn't the Ritalin controlling the impulsivity and the temper tantrums?

We continued on for many more weeks in our confusion, baffled by the behaviors of our little six year old until, finally, we reached the point of despair.

Instead of calling the pediatrician for an examination, I requested an appointment to go in for a consultation. After hearing our latest list of problems, the doctor's first suggestion was to increase Ryan's medication, to which I readily agreed. I then asked the doctor about the possibility of having Ryan examined by a neurologist, but the pediatrician explained that it would, in his opinion, really be unnecessary. After all, he reasoned, in the absence of a seizure disorder, a neurologist's treatment of Ryan would be exactly the same as he, the pediatrician, was already providing. He did say that we were completely free to consult a neurologist on our own, if we so desired, and he even offered to recommend one, but he added that our insurance company would not pay for the visit without his authorization of the referral. He mentioned that a neurological examination would probably be expensive, but that it might very well be worth our peace of mind to have a second opinion.

"Please doctor," I pleaded. "If it were your child and he was suffering with a heart problem, I'm sure you would want him evaluated by a specialist in cardiology. Well, our son has a neurological problem. Please," I asked imploringly, "on the slightest chance that we may have missed something, won't you please reconsider and authorize us to have Ryan examined by a neurologist?" Somehow, by the end of the consultation, the doctor's opinion had softened and he had agreed to authorize one visit to a pediatric neurologist.

Our local medical group contracts for neurological services with a neurologist from one of the large university hospitals in Los Angeles. The specialist comes to our area on a periodic basis and sees patients at one of our local community hospitals. Ryan's pediatrician arranged an appointment for us to take Ryan in during the neurologist's next visit to our area, and Jim arranged a special day off from work in order to go with us.

Jim and I entered the examination room with nervous anticipation and high hopes that this specialist in neurological disorders would be able to offer us some answers to our difficult situation and help for our little boy's problems.

The doctor was very direct in his approach and went quickly to work. Ryan, who was sitting on an examining table, was asked to hold both of his hands up flat, then asked to turn them over, this time palms facing upward. He was asked to get off the table and to hop across the floor, first on one leg, and then on the other. The doctor helped him back on the table and tapped his knees with a small gavel to check his reflexes. He then shined a light in both of Ryan's eyes asking him to follow the light as he moved it around. The entire exam took less than ten minutes.

The doctor began to speak as he moved toward the door. "Mr. and Mrs. Hughes, he began, your son has what is known as Attention Deficit Disorder with Hyperactivity. And he then continued on to describe the symptoms of ADDH. We could tell that he was ready to leave the room and I suddenly spurted out, "But what about the babbling spells he's been having?" "What babbling spells," he asked?"

I began to describe the erratic "babbling" episodes that Ryan had been having for the past two years, which was our primary reason for being in his office in the first place. I began by explaining that these were periods of time when he would seem to lose all touch with the world around him. He would laugh and babble and have a glazed look in his eyes. He would throw his body around, either becoming limp when picked up or sometimes very stiff and rigid. When the episodes would be over, never lasting more than five to ten minutes, he would act normal again, never seeming to know what had happened. During these episodes we would try to talk to him, looking directly into his little eyes, but there was no recognition. We were unable to get through to him.

The neurologist listened as Jim and I described our concerns. He concluded that the symptoms we described were unusual, but he assured us he was confident that it was not a seizure disorder of any type and once again he turned to leave. "But what about another EEG," I asked hastily. "Should he have another EEG done," I questioned? "Yes, it might be a good idea to get one done periodically," he said. "Just be glad, Mr. and Mrs. Hughes," he continued in a patronizing tone, "that we now have medication to help these kids. Twenty years ago there was nothing to help children with this problem. I'll get a letter off to your doctor regarding my findings."

Jim and I left the hospital feeling very desolate and discouraged. We slowly drove the few miles back home, in total silence, contemplating how much longer we could face life with this little "Jekyll and Hyde" and wondering if things would ever be normal for our family. We never mentioned to Ryan's pediatrician the results of the visit with the "specialist," remembering his hesitation to authorize the visit in the first place, and he never mentioned it to us.

Ryan's transitional year in school turned out to be

a huge success and he was promoted to a full year of first grade with flying colors! The school assessment team recommended that Ryan continue with time in the resource room again the following year, with the tutor concentrating on helping his handwriting, his self-esteem and, especially, his social behavior.

One of the highlights of the year was Ryan's success in baseball! Ryan's coach was impressed with Ryan's "strong arm" and gave him a chance to play third base all season. During one afternoon game, Ryan surprised everyone by making a Triple Play all by himself!

But still hanging over our heads was our son's erratic, unpredictable and impulsive behavior. Of equal concern was Ryan's growth. An x-ray of Ryan's hand done earlier in the year revealed that his bone age was approximately two years behind his chronological age. Although he posted a slight bit of growth at each three month check-up, he was still not "on" the pediatrician's growth chart for either height or weight.

Was this from the Ritalin? It was a strong possibility, but we knew that taking him off the medication was not something we could consider at that point. Just seeing his violent, explosive behavior when the pills were wearing off gave justification to continuing the medication.

We had experimented with the drug Dexedrine, also a psychostimulant medication, but did not get the same beneficial results we did with Ritalin, so we continued on with efforts to alter Ryan's mealtimes when he might be under less effect of the pills and more willing to eat. But on most days there was no food that could elicit a happy response from Ryan. Eating was his least favorite thing to do. It would break my heart to finish my own lunch or dinner and realize that he had not even taken a bite of his.

There were many, many days that grace from above was the only thing that got me through the day. I felt tremendous love and devotion for this little child of mine, yet nothing that I tried to do seemed to help except giving him those stupid little pills. I hated those pills! I agonized over those pills! Yet I knew that as surely as the diabetic needed insulin, my little Ryan needed this medical intervention to allow him to be a "normal" child.

I had started attending a support group for parents called the California Association of Neurologically Handicapped Children. It was still very difficult for me to admit that Ryan was neurologically handicapped but I was increasingly aware of how different he was from other children. I was hungry for information on Attention Deficit Disorder and hyperactivity but found that most of the books printed were several years old and many did not have current or up-to-date information.

I wrote to CIBA, the manufacturer of Ritalin, in an effort to learn more about the drug and perhaps any studies they may have conducted showing the effects of long-term usage. Because Ritalin was not recommended for usage in children under the age of six, I was interested in any information they could provide, as Ryan had started on their product at the age of three. But the company's representative sent a written reply stating that there was no information about the drug available for distribution to the general public. They did, however, enclose the same pamphlet that our first pediatrician had given us when telling us that Ryan had Minimal Brain

Dysfunction, only the title on the brochure they sent had been changed to reflect the new name, Attention Deficit Disorder.

Jim, too, had begun to seek information on these disorders by attending any conferences or workshops he could find relating to special education. He enrolled in a class at a nearby university on "Exceptional Children," and as part of an assigned project, Jim and I presented a talk on our experiences of being parents of an "exceptional child." It somehow helped to share our feelings to that group of teachers — to let them know how we as parents felt in trying to cope with a disorder that had the power to wreak such havoc on our family life and to push our parental capacities to the limit.

I knew that there must be other mothers out there just like me who needed someone to talk to. I thought seriously of starting a local support group for mothers of hyperactive kids, but I didn't have the energy or the self-confidence that I could offer help to anyone else. I was hurting too much myself. But when I did learn of other mothers with children who had similar problems, I would always invite them over for coffee and we would share our experiences. Yet I never met anyone who had a six year old that was still wetting his pants (daytime only), spitting and running out in front of cars.

Something inside of me kept saying, "there's an answer for this." Yet each corner that I turned seemed to make the hope of an answer less and less likely.

Chapter 11
All Star Boy

First grade was a fun year for Ryan. The transition year had been just what he needed to gain growing time emotionally and he entered school that year with enthusiasm and lots of confidence. He once again had the same first- grade teacher and even the same classroom as he had during the first- grade portion of the transition year.

I must admit I was more than a little nervous. The first week of school the teacher called to tell me that Ryan had broken another student's eyeglasses. It seemed that the other student had taken them off on the playground and laid them down on the pavement providing Ryan with just enough temptation to pick them up and see how far in the air they would go!

During the school's open house night, I walked into the classroom and overheard another mother asking the teacher where Ryan Hughes' seat was located. My first impulse was to turn the other way. I was certain that this mother had already heard about Ryan and his Dennis the Menace shenanigans and that she was wanting to make sure her child wasn't assigned the seat next to him. When the teacher introduced me to the inquiring mom I learned that her daughter was really quite taken by Ryan and had requested that her mother have a chance to meet his mother! Ryan made several friends that year, and he was even invited to a couple of birthday parties — a first for him!

Academically, Ryan did exceptionally well that year. His handwriting and fine motor skills continued to be his weakest area but he learned to read and he showed a genuine interest in learning. Although his work was progressing nicely, Ryan's behavior was still a problem at school. The teacher began to send home "behavior notes" daily, and she would write down specific problems that he had that day. Spitting on the playground, knocking down other students, hitting, biting and shoving were a few of the problems she was dealing with.

He had also started showing some behaviors which were new, and strange. For several months he had what seemed to be a habit of wiping his hair out of his eyes, yet his hair was not even long enough to be in his eyes. When we questioned him about it, he had no explanation for why he did it, and he wasn't even aware he had been doing it. He also had begun to stick his tongue out at people. These "habits" lasted several months and then went away. We never made a big deal about them and never really gave much thought to them. But the spitting was still causing us a lot of worry. He would spit on other people, sometimes at strangers in a store. And then he would start laughing and "babbling" as we called it.

Once again the subject of Tourette syndrome had been brought to our attention. In one of the recent teacher conferences that Jim had attended there was a doctor from the City of Hope Medical Center in Los Angeles who had done a presentation on Tourette syndrome. He had mentioned that one of the symptoms or "tics," as he called them, involved in the disorder was spitting. Jim had queried the doctor further after the meeting thinking that perhaps this might be a clue to the spitting problem. On our next visit to the psychologist we asked if he thought Ryan's spitting might be a symptom of Tourette syndrome and he said that he did not think so. But he did advise that he found Ryan's problems to be somewhat complex and he recommended that we consult a pediatric psychiatrist.

Because our insurance program is a health maintenance organization we are not permitted to go to any doctor outside our local medical group without prior authorization from our pediatrician. I called Ryan's doctor to discuss in detail some of the problems we were having and to get a referral to a child psychiatrist. He recommended a local doctor and we arranged for our first appointment. We talked openly and freely about all of Ryan's behaviors, about our home and family life, and the various behavior modification programs we had been using with Ryan. After meeting with us two or three times, the psychiatrist concluded that we were doing all of the "right" things with Ryan and that it would not be beneficial to enter into any long-term therapy. He suggested that we come in for visits on an "as needed" basis. We were disappointed that he offered nothing new as far as help or interventions, but were very grateful that he was honest in not bringing us in for lengthy and costly therapy that might not be helpful.

Indeed, we had tried to do all of the "right" things. We studied information on various behavior modification techniques and tried several different programs at home. We continually praised Ryan's efforts and made a big deal out of any successes that he had. We tried to reward the good instead of dwelling on the bad. But there were many, many days that we failed miserably. We yelled, we screamed, we threatened, we pleaded, we spanked, we took away privileges and we stripped his room of all toys. There were days when exhaustion and despair were rampant, but, always, there was love for this little child of ours who we couldn't understand. There was never a day that Ryan was not reminded many times of our love for him, and hugs and kisses flowed freely, even after frustrating episodes.

Ryan's dosage of Ritalin had risen to sixty milligrams per day, a very large daily dosage for a child his age, and according to the pediatrician, the maximum dose for his weight, which was approximately forty pounds. We had tried during the summer months before school started to give him Cylert, but after only several days he developed a severe headache with violent vomiting. He became lethargic and pale and we took him to the emergency room for treatment. It is still not clear if the medication caused the episode; however, we discontinued the Cylert after that incident and have never tried it since.

It was during this year that I first heard Ryan say a curse word. I decided that I would "nip it in the bud" and I admonished him harshly, explaining emphatically to him that we did not use words like that in our home and that his dad and I would not permit him to use that language. I was sure he had heard it on the playground at school. I was shocked, when a few days later, I heard

Ryan repeat several curse words over and over again. When I attempted to reprimand him the words came louder and more frequently. I spanked him hard and put him in the time-out room, but it did no good. The cursing continued, although it was sporadic in nature, and completely unpredictable.

From that day on, periodically, for no reason at all, Ryan would start uttering a series of four-letter words and would repeat them over and over. Many times these "favorite" words would be accompanied by a stupid kind of laugh, much like the laugh he had when he began the "babbling" at the age of three. There were a few times when I could distract him or get him to stop, but most of the time nothing that Jim or I could do would help. It was as if it just had to run its course or that he had to get it out of his system. A few times I found the words written on pieces of paper around the house. He had spelled the words as they sounded phonetically, and sometimes the letters were written backwards.

Any doubts that I may have had about Ryan's ability to "prevent" saying the words were quickly erased the night that I heard him cursing in his sleep. It was not unusual for him to talk or yell out while asleep; however, this particular night, he was having a conversation with someone. During the conversation he would repeat four or five curse words, in a string, over and over. Then he would resume with the conversation as if nothing had happened. This happened several times throughout the episode and Ryan, still asleep, had absolutely no knowledge that his dad and I were listening outside his door.

From then on, Jim and I tried ignoring the outbursts,

but it didn't seem to matter if we reacted to them or remained silent. This type of behavior was extremely distressing, especially when it happened in a public setting or at church.

It was also about this time that he started another peculiar "habit." He was constantly tugging and pulling his pants up — even if they didn't need it! This habit lasted several months. It didn't matter what he was wearing, shorts or jeans, loose or tight; he was constantly going through the motion of pulling up his pants. It was particularly noticeable when he was on the ball field. But we tried to ignore it. We felt that Ryan had enough problems without nagging him about something that was causing no one any harm.

Along with the arrival of spring came the advent of Little League season and Ryan was thrilled to be playing baseball again. He had a really good year playing third base and he even had the opportunity to pitch in several games. At the end of the season Ryan was selected to be on the All Star Team and his dad and I were bursting with pride when his name was announced on the loudspeaker and he ran onto the field to accept his All Star hat. It had been his first year on a farm division team and being chosen for the All Star team was a great honor.

Although his individual team did not fare well in the post-season competition, just getting to play and being a part of the team was a tremendous boost for Ryan. The boys were honored with black jackets that noted their All Star achievement on the back, and he wore that jacket to bed the first few nights, afraid that if he took it off it would disappear. Ryan's success in baseball meant more to him than many people may have imagined. Finally, there was something he was good at! Instead of hearing criticisms all the time, he was being praised. He loved having the other boys' parents yell his name at the games and cheer for him, although he coyly pretended not to notice. We whole heartedly encouraged him in his efforts to play baseball and his dad and I both have sat through hundreds of hours of games and practices, thoroughly enjoying every minute of watching him play.

It was during this year that our family had an opportunity to buy a beautiful home in a small community just twenty miles southeast of where we were living. Both Ryan and Julie were excited about the upcoming move and especially about getting a larger new house with a community pool! A brand-new elementary school just down at the end of our street was set to open in September and Ryan was excited that he would be able to walk to his new school.

Ryan had done so well with his repeat of first grade that the school assessment team at his previous school was hard pressed in writing his IEP (individualized education plan) or to recommend his continuance in the resource program for the following year. Although his test scores had come up considerably, thanks to the "extra" year of instruction and the special tutoring he had received, the IEP team still felt that Ryan, because of his ongoing medical and behavior problems, was at extremely high risk for learning disabilities.

It was the IEP team's recommendation that he remain in the resource program in his new school district and that his tutoring time be centered around his fine motor difficulties and his poor handwriting. We were extremely grateful for all of the wonderful help and support Ryan's previous teachers had given him, and we were looking forward to settling into our new home and getting the children enrolled in their new schools.

Chapter 12
The Agony of Defeat

Several weeks before school was to start I met with the special education director of our new school district in order to introduce myself and to ask their procedure in enrolling Ryan in their special education resource program. She explained that as soon as they received a copy of the IEP that had been written by Ryan's previous school district, that they would review the district's recommendations, and then have thirty days to accept or reject the placement.

I then phoned the principal of Ryan's new school to make her aware of Ryan's particular problems and to ask her assistance in assigning him to a teacher who might be best suited for children with Attention Deficit Disorder. She assured me that she would do her best and that Ryan's tutoring would begin as soon as school started and continue until the district had a chance to review his placement. Everything sounded in order to me and I felt very secure that I had done all that I could possibly do to make the transition to the new school a smooth one both for Ryan and for the district. When I received a notice of an IEP meeting just a few weeks later I didn't give it a second thought. Just a formality, I thought to myself. I concluded that I would probably have to sign the paperwork again insofar that it was a new district. The notice I received concerning the upcoming meeting stated that a school administrator was to be present, along with the classroom teacher and the school nurse. Although I had been through several IEP meetings before with no problems whatsoever, for some unknown reason I always felt somewhat intimidated by these semiformal sessions.

The meeting began at two-fifteen that afternoon. Those present included the school principal, special education director, resource room teacher (tutor), and the school nurse. After the usual introductions, the resource room teacher began to read her observations and recommendations for Ryan's placement: Ryan's behavior is acceptable at most times. Ryan's handwriting needs improvement. Ryan's teacher reports that his academic work is satisfactory at this time. His behavior is also acceptable. Ryan's handwriting is more legible when he takes his time. He reverses letters fairly often. It is recommended that Ryan continue to do all academic work in the regular classroom at this time. His teacher will need to remind Ryan to take his time when doing handwriting so that it is neater. Discharge from the RSP program recommended.

I couldn't believe what I was hearing! A relatively new teacher, not long out of college, had decided that Ryan did not need any special help and she had recommended to the special education director and the principal that he be dismissed from the resource tutoring program!

I sat there in silence for a few long seconds, stunned by their unexpected proposal. I then asked the principal

70

where Ryan's classroom teacher was, and why she was not present at the meeting, as my notice had indicated. The principal mentioned that she thought the teacher was planning to come to the meeting and was not sure why she had been unable to attend. I then asked the resource specialist if she had spoken with Ryan's teacher to determine how he was doing in class, and she said that they both had been very busy with the starting of school, but that she did talk with the teacher briefly in passing just a couple of days earlier. I began to explain about Ryan's previous academic problems and our concerns that he might not do as well as he had the previous year, as it had actually been a "repeat" of first grade. I expressed concern that this would be the first year that he would have to prove himself in the classroom with a new teacher and new material and I emphasized his problems with attention and behavior.

Although the school officials listened patiently as I described Ryan's academic and medical history, and the reasons that the previous school district had decided to continue his placement in the special education program, it seemed that their decision had been finalized. The school administrators then offered me a form to sign that would release Ryan from the special education program as they had recommended. I could feel myself begin to shake inwardly as I realized that I, a parent alone, was outnumbered and that the pressure was on me to sign the form. But thank heaven my mouth took over when my brain failed and I heard myself asking for time to think it over and discuss it with my husband before signing.

Jim and I both knew how very difficult it was to get children with Attention Deficit Disorder "qualified" for special help in the public schools. Because funds are so very limited, the state has a very strict criterium that requires that a child must show a two- grade discrepancy between his test scores and ability before qualifying for any special tutoring help. Many times, throughout Jim's twenty years of teaching experience, we had seen children have to struggle through several years of failure until they were so far behind that they finally could qualify for extra help under the state's guidelines. We didn't want that to happen to Ryan. It only made sense to us to help him *before* he fell behind, especially in view of his potential for learning disabilities associated with the Attention Deficit Disorder.

But what was even more disturbing to us was the fact that a relatively inexperienced teacher could make such a critical decision about a child that she had seen only fifteen minutes a day for less than two weeks! Also, after talking with the classroom teacher, we learned that she had never actually had a formal meeting with the tutor about Ryan, but just as the resource teacher had said, they had discussed his problems briefly while passing through the school one day. Surely our son's academic placement deserved more consideration than this!

I made another appointment with the special education director and respectfully requested that they reconsider refusing Ryan's placement in their resource program. I explained to her that Jim and I could not, in good conscience, agree to remove him from the program and that we would like to be provided with a copy of our parental rights regarding the special education program. She was very gracious but did not offer us much encouragement. She did say, however, that she would once again talk it over with the principal and the school psychologist.

My next phone call was to the school psychologist. I provided him with copies of the psychological report from the previous school district and also with a letter from Ryan's pediatrician outlining Ryan's medical background and continued need for special education services. It was a few days later that I received notice of the school district's decision to conduct their own diagnostic testing to determine if Ryan would qualify for placement in their special education program. I signed, without hesitation, the permission form to allow the testing to begin.

It was an anxious time waiting for their results. We did not know what to expect and did not want the situation to turn into an "us against them" situation. Still, we had resolved in our minds that we KNEW our little boy. We had been living and suffering with his disabilities for the past seven years, yet a small group of strangers who had seen him briefly for only a few weeks were making decisions that would affect the rest of his academic life! We had emphasized to the district officials that they were seeing Ryan under the effect of sixty milligrams of Ritalin a day. They were seeing him at his "best"! Jim and I were sure they didn't know the real Ryan yet, although as the days went on, notes from the classroom teacher revealed that she was beginning to see many problems surface.

It was nearly a month later that I received notice from the district that their testing had been completed and that another IEP meeting would be held. I requested a copy of the psychologist's report in writing, *before* the meeting, as I wanted to be prepared for whatever position the district might take. Jim and I were so firm in our belief for Ryan's need for special help that we were prepared to appeal to the state department of education if necessary to exercise our right to a "fair hearing."

The school district's test results of Ryan's work showed a reduction in test scores from the previous year's tests that had been done in the other district. In addition, Ryan showed a severe discrepancy in his test scores between ability and achievement in the mathematics area. He also evidenced a processing disorder in attention. It was now the recommendation by the psychologist and the rest of the IEP team that Ryan be allowed to continue in the special education resource program and that he continue to receive psychiatric and psychological intervention.

We were greatly relieved that Ryan was going to continue to be afforded some extra help and we were very impressed with the school officials willingness to reconsider Ryan's placement and pursue the matter with further testing.

As I was leaving the meeting, the school nurse, a sympathetic and kind lady, pulled me aside and asked if she might speak with me privately for a minute. "Mrs. Hughes," she began, "perhaps I shouldn't mention this, but I have listened to you describe Ryan's behavior and the episodes he is having with spitting and swearing. Have you ever considered that he may possibly have Tourette syndrome?" I told her that, yes, we had thought of that, but that Ryan's psychologist had said that the spitting was not caused by Tourette syndrome. She then

74

very graciously offered me a paper with a phone number of a doctor at the City of Hope Medical Center in Los Angeles who specializes in children with that disorder. She encouraged me to call them and to request their literature. I thanked her for her help and a few days later called the number and requested some information.

When the literature from the City of Hope Medical Center arrived, I read with much interest some of the symptoms and diagnostic criteria of Tourette syndrome. Vocal or motor tics were the most common. But Ryan didn't have any "tics," or so I thought. As I read further I discovered that "tics" were not just jerking and twitching movements as I had previously thought. Some examples of motor tics were: "hair out of the eyes tic" and "tugging at the clothing" and "pulling up the socks." Ryan had been doing all of those things off and on for the past year and a half! Vocal tics were described as "grunting, spitting, or other vocal noises." I wondered if perhaps "babbling" might also be considered a tic.

I read in amazement the descriptions of the typical Tourette patient: "Jekyll & Hyde personality, can't take no for an answer, compulsive swearing, explosive, hurts animals or parents. Reading that brochure was like reading a book about Ryan! So many of those things seemed to describe him perfectly! I made copies of the brochure and made an appointment with Ryan's pediatrician to discuss my findings with him.

Ryan's doctor read with interest the information on Tourette syndrome that I provided. He agreed that Tourette syndrome in Ryan was certainly an area to be investigated. But when I asked if he would refer us to the City of Hope Medical Center, in order that our insurance

nervous system. Things at this time weren't going too well, by any means, but we did see some slight improvement.

It was one day in the spring when a neighbor called to tell me that she had seen an article in the Los Angeles Times asking for eight year old hyperactive boys to participate in a research study program. The studies were to be done at the National Center for Hyperactive Children, about thirty miles from our home and would involve a series of eight visits. In exchange for the child's participation, the family would receive free advice and psychological recommendations from the doctor, who, as the head of the clinic, had vast experience in dealing with hyperactive children. Jim and I had heard of the doctor and his fine reputation previously, and his work had been featured on the ABC television program, 20/20, in August 1987.

After requesting and receiving information about the research project we decided to submit Ryan's application for two reasons. One reason was to contribute to the doctor's research studies. Certainly our son, with his severe hyperactivity, would be a choice model for the research and possibly someday the doctors and researchers could find a cause and cure for this bizarre behavioral disorder. Also, Jim and I hoped that this doctor would openly share his expertise with us and perhaps offer some new suggestions for Ryan's difficult problems.

There was to be no cost involved for the program (and no authorization needed from our pediatrician), and certainly the thirty minute drive from home for only eight sessions would be well worth having this excellent physician's opinion.

Admission to the research project was done very selectively. Before being allowed to come for the first visit we were screened carefully over the phone by the doctor's assistant. We were then mailed information sheets to fill out and we waited anxiously to see if we would be allowed to proceed to the next step. We were called again by the assistant within a few weeks time, and were asked to come into the clinic and to fill out a new series of questionnaires. It was quite a lengthy assortment of questions as I remember. The inquiries were specific and covered in complete detail every facet of the child's history and behavior patterns and also information about each of us parents! A few more weeks had passed when we finally received notice that Ryan had been accepted into the program. We were to meet with the doctor at our next visit.

Jim and I went together to the appointment, and we listened attentively as this well-known and nationally respected doctor sat and talked with us for over an hour and a half. He queried us more specifically about our answers on the questionnaires, pressing us further for details and for every bit and piece of information we could provide regarding the behavior of our hyperactive son. It seemed that there was no stone left unturned. He made notes of all of our answers and, after the ninety minute session was through, he put his pen down on the desk and slowly began to offer his opinion.

I felt warm tears begin to sting my eyes and cheeks as the doctor started to speak. "Mr. and Mrs. Hughes," he began, " I am so very sorry to tell you this, but I will not be able to continue to include Ryan in our research program. You see, he said sympathetically, our research is for eight year old boys who have only Attention Deficit Disorder with hyperactivity. We cannot accept children with any other types of disorders as it would negate or invalidate our research."

He continued by saying, "It is evident to me, Mr. and Mrs. Hughes, that Ryan is most probably suffering from a neurological disorder known as Tourette syndrome. In addition, I feel that it is imperative that he has a thorough neurological workup by a pediatric neurologist in order to rule out any underlying seizure disorder. I would also encourage you to have another EEG done as soon as possible and I would recommend that you go to a doctor who specializes in these types of problems. I would be happy to recommend a doctor at the Neuropsychiatric Department at UCLA or at the City of Hope Medical Center where they are doing a lot of work with Tourette syndrome. I also feel that your son has a separation anxiety disorder, a conduct disorder, and several phobias." In conclusion, the doctor advised that 60 milligrams of Ritalin was, in his opinion, entirely too much medication, and that it was imperative to have Ryan re-evaluated as he was by all means suffering from more than just hyperactivity.

Words cannot describe my feelings as we made our way through the heavy freeway traffic back home. What were we going to do? There was no way that we could go to the clinics at UCLA or at the City of Hope Medical Center on our own! We were sure those clinics would be far too expensive for us to afford.

We began by calling our pediatrician, the doctor who must authorize any referrals outside of our local clinic. After sharing the hyperactivity specialist's findings with him, he was very sympathetic and said that he was sure that it wouldn't be necessary for us to go all the way to UCLA or the City of Hope Medical Center. He was confident that everything could be handled locally and he continued on to say that if it proved necessary, he could refer us to a local neurologist. But before doing that, however, he would order another EEG. He then advised us to make another appointment with Ryan's psychiatrist to let him know of the findings from the hyperactivity specialist.

When I called the psychiatrist to tell him of this new development, he expressed surprise that the specialist would suggest the possibility of Tourette syndrome. "I know I'm just a small town doctor up against the big city specialist," he said wryly, "but I just don't see Tourette syndrome in your son!" I asked if perhaps he and Ryan's pediatrician could call the doctor at City of Hope Hospital and confer with him about the possibility of Tourettes. He didn't answer my question but, instead, began to explain that he had never observed any Tourette symptoms during his visits with Ryan. He did agree, however, that another EEG was in order.

Ryan's second EEG was done a short time after our conversation with the psychiatrist and it too came back normal. The hyperactivity specialist had warned us that a normal EEG was not concrete evidence that there was not an underlying seizure disorder and that we should insist on having a neurological workup done. He had explained that there are some seizure disorders that are so deep in the brain that they cannot be detected by the superficial tracings of a standard EEG. He had encouraged us to persist in seeking a referral for a complete neurological evaluation. Despite his recommendation, when the second EEG came back normal, Jim and I were reluctant to press the pediatrician for the neurological referral, especially since the psychiatrist was still denying the evidence of Tourette syndrome.

Ryan's psychiatrist had mentioned to us several months previously the possibility of hospitalizing Ryan in the children's ward of the local mental health hospital for observation. We were totally against hospitalization, especially when we were told that we could not stay with him, but things were getting much, much worse and we were at our wits' end. At our next visit, instead of hospitalization, as we feared, the doctor offered adding a new drug to be taken along with the Ritalin. Ryan was started on the drug Stelazine (a major tranquilizer) and it seemed for a short while that he was doing a little bit better. But the improvement didn't last long. In desperation I called the psychiatrist again.

"Please help," I pleaded. "Ryan is worse! What can we do?" "Let's add some Benadryl to the Stelazine and the Ritalin," he offered. "Sometimes Benadryl helps to calm these kids down. Let me know how it goes." I sat, in disbelief, for a few minutes, holding the phone receiver in my hand, the dial tone urging me to hang up. At that moment, I felt numb all over. I knew with every sense of my being that this just wasn't right. I was very familiar with the allergy drug Benadryl and its side effect of causing drowsiness. But to add that drug to the two powerful drugs that Ryan was already taking, just to make him drowsy, was more than I could accept.

I picked up the phone again and this time dialed information. "May I have the number of the City of Hope

Medical Center please?," I asked the operator, choking back the tears. When the receptionist at the hospital answered, I asked for the Tourette Syndrome Clinic and I was shocked when the doctor himself answered the phone. I introduced myself and began to give him a brief history about Ryan. He asked me several questions and said that it sounded very probable that Ryan did indeed have several symptoms associated with Tourette syndrome.

"But he doesn't twitch and jerk," I said. "Can he still have Tourette syndrome if he doesn't do that," I asked? He assured me that, "Yes, sometimes the tics are mostly vocal." "Also," I cautioned, "the Ritalin seems to stop the swearing, the spitting and the screaming out. Is that possible?" I continued. "It does happen in some cases," he said.

The doctor continued on to say that we should make an appointment to bring Ryan into the clinic to be evaluated, but unfortunately they were so heavily booked that it would be at least several months before they could fit us in.

The doctor must have sensed my despair. "I don't think you can wait that long can you," he asked knowingly. "No sir," I replied. "I don't believe we can." "Just a minute, Mrs. Hughes," he said, "I think you should come in as soon as possible. I'll have my secretary work you in. I'll try to get you in to see us within the next two weeks."

I couldn't wait for Jim to get home from work to tell him the news! This well-known doctor at the City of Hope Medical Center also seemed to think that Ryan might have Tourette syndrome! I hadn't even mentioned to him that the hyperactivity specialist had suggested it too!

While we waited for our upcoming appointment, we continued Ryan's medication just as it had been previously with the Stelazine and Ritalin. We did not add the Benadryl as Ryan's psychiatrist had suggested, but waited patiently for our appointment, hoping that somehow, someway, someone could provide us with the help that we so desperately needed.

Chapter 13
Hope

A few days after my conversation with the doctor at the City of Hope Medical Center we received a large packet of papers, including exhaustive questionnaires that were to be filled out, in much detail, by each of the four of us. We were instructed to bring our questionnaires with us to the first appointment and to be at the hospital by eight-thirty that morning in order to have blood work done on Jim, myself, and Ryan. We were told that it was to be a fasting blood test and that none of us were to eat after midnight the night before.

Our home is located about sixty-five miles north of the hospital and getting there by eight-thirty in the morning would put us right in the middle of heavy rush hour traffic going through the center of Los Angeles. We decided that instead of fighting nearly two hours of stop-and-go traffic on the freeway we would travel down the night before and stay in a motel close by the hospital.

We were fortunate to find a beautiful brand new hotel just several miles away that accepted our fifty percent discount coupon from the teacher's association, and it also offered a beautiful pool where Jim and I could relax and where Ryan could splash and swim. We had a

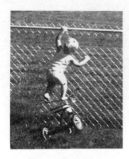 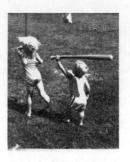

Ryan over the
backyard fence

After his sister
with a bat

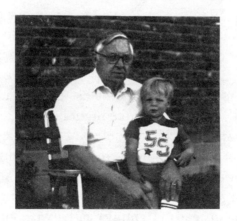

Ryan with Papaw Hughes

photo 1

Ihave q villianit is teret syndrom
I dont like it causeit Makes
youdoStuff rong
todayitmade me hitPeoPle
I dont likeitwhen itmakes
me throw thing

Ryan's dyslexic handwriting at 9 years of age
I have a villian - it is Tourette syndrome
I don't like it cause it makes you do stuff wrong
Today it made me hit people
I don't like it when it makes me throw things

I dont like it when it makes
me say Bad wordsI wishI
wouldenthave it soI could
Play more and have morefun

I don't like it when it makes
me say bad words I wish I
wouldn't have it so I could
play more and have more fun

R Yq

1 234 56 < 8 90 1)£|9|4|5|6|

Ryan's name and numbers

photo 2

fun evening together and we were happy to be only five minutes away when time came to leave for the hospital early the next morning.

Ryan had only had blood drawn twice before and both times had proven to be quite an experience. He had a real phobia about needles and he often worked himself up into a faint just thinking about getting a blood test, or a shot. We didn't tell him until we got to the hospital that morning that we all were going to have our blood tested, and just learning that Mom and Dad were having blood tests too seemed to help Ryan accept the inevitable. I volunteered to go first thinking that I could show Ryan what a cinch it was and possibly be able to help relieve his worries.

As I sat down in the chair the technician explained that they would be drawing seven tubes of blood from each of us and she began dutifully drawing the first tube. She had just started to draw the fourth tube of blood when I began to feel-light headed. By the time she had started to draw the fifth tube I had fainted and awakened to find the room full of doctors and nurses! They explained that my blood pressure was quite low and that they were going to take me to the recovery room for a while for observation.

How embarrassing, I thought to myself. I was still feeling a little weak and was in a sort of "fog," and the next thing I knew, they were wheeling me right out the door in front of Ryan! The poor little fellow really panicked when he saw his brave Mom being carted out of the lab on a gurney, ghastly pale and looking like death warmed over.

The nurses tried to reassure Ryan that I was fine and

that he would be, too, but he would have no part of it. When the technician tried to take his hand to lead him into the lab for his blood test, he broke away and began running through the hospital. He dashed through the waiting room and right out the front door of the hospital with his father and the lab technician in hot pursuit! He continued to run, racing right out into the crowded parking lot and dodging the cars and people who were watching with bewilderment. Fortunately, the hospital security guard saw Jim frantically yelling and trying to catch up to the child with the legs that were traveling faster than the speed of sound. With the guard's help Jim was able to capture Ryan and to carry the kicking and screaming fugitive back into the hospital!

It took six adults, including two strong men, to hold him down, but a short time later, the hospital staff emerged victorious with seven full tubes of blood! Ryan was fine after the needle had been inserted and was even able to go out and have a nice big breakfast before his appointment with the doctor later that afternoon. As for me, I learned to never have blood drawn after fasting for more than sixteen hours and to never volunteer to be a role model when having a blood test!

"I heard you had a little trouble this morning," said the doctor as we settled in our chairs in the small examining room. Actually, I was thinking to myself, everything was running pretty true to form for the Hughes family. It seemed that nothing ever ran smoothly for us with Ryan's constant escapades and perpetual motion.

The doctor was a kind man who seemed to have a sympathetic and gentle spirit. We sat quietly for quite some time as he poured over the volume of information in the questionnaire forms we had completed and brought in with us. Then his questioning began.

The doctor listened patiently as we explained our answers in more detail and he pressed for more and more information concerning Ryan's past history and behavior problems. He wrote down pages and pages of notes riddled with symbols that were foreign to me. There were lots of questions about mine and Jim's backgrounds and our behaviors and circumstances throughout childhood and adolescence. When he finished, I was sure that there was nothing else about any of the three of us left to reveal.

After what seemed like hours, this soft-spoken and highly respected doctor began to offer his opinion. "Ryan has a classical, full-blown case of Tourette syndrome," he began forthrightly. He then cited many of the behaviors that we had thought of as habits to actually be "tics," all common for the neurological disorder. The spitting, cursing, and screaming out loud and the "babbling" were all considered to be "vocal tics," while the "hair out of the eyes, pulling up the socks, and tugging at the clothing" were all considered to be motor tics. Also present were the obsessive-compulsive behaviors that Ryan had exhibited and the perseveration, or the inability to give up a certain thought.

The doctor explained that Attention Deficit Disorder with hyperactivity is closely linked with Tourette syndrome, often being one of the first manifestations of the disorder. He continued to say that Attention Deficit Disorder usually precedes the onset of motor and vocal tics by an average of two and one-half years. This was certainly the case in Ryan's situation as the hyperactivity was evident two to three years before the spitting and cursing began. Other manifestations of Tourettes such as learning disabilities, dyslexia, and especially problems with math and handwriting were also described. Ryan continues, even now, to have problems with handwriting and math and even at the age of nine still reverses some letters and words!

The doctor explained that conduct and discipline problems are evident in thirty-five percent of patients with Tourette syndrome. Symptoms such as having a short temper, everything being a confrontation, compulsively picking on siblings, getting into fights, inappropriate shouting, inability to take responsibility for his own actions, Jekyll and Hyde personality, and being abusive to pets and sometimes even to parents were all behaviors that we had been suffering through with Ryan for years, yet all typical behaviors in children with Tourette syndrome!

Also common with this disorder were panic attacks and phobias. Ryan had displayed a phobia of insects for the past several years and just the thought of a needle (blood test) or getting a splinter out of his finger would cause him to get short of breath, break out in a sweat and faint! He also had a phobia about being in a room alone and would often panic if he looked up and discovered that one of us had walked out and left him for even just a few minutes!

The doctor spent quite some time explaining the symptoms and treatment of Tourette syndrome with us. He explained that Stelazine was not the first drug of choice but because Ryan was already on a regimen of

Stelazine and Ritalin we could continue on with it, adding a dosage of Prozac to try to help stabilize his behavior and control the tics. We were to keep in touch with him by phone and to return in six weeks for another follow-up visit.

As the three of us left the hospital hand in hand I was bursting with joy on the inside. I wanted to shout to the top of my lungs to everyone I passed, "Our son has Tourette syndrome and it's NOT our fault. His behavior is NOT OUR FAULT OR HIS FAULT!" For the first time in nine years we finally had an explanation for all of the miseries and torturous days that we had endured. There was finally a name for the disease that had robbed our family of the privilege of sharing a normal life together.

Surprisingly, I was not bitter, as one might expect, nor was I angry at the psychiatrist who had persisted in his ignorance to misdiagnose, despite the obvious symptoms. At that moment I felt only relief and satisfaction that a correct diagnosis had been reached and confirmed by one of the top specialists in the field. I felt tremendously blessed that finally we were being given not only information, but hope that our future with Ryan might not be totally disastrous!

It was several days before reality sank in and I began to deal with the knowledge that my son indeed had a neurological handicap called Tourette syndrome and that it wasn't such a wonderful thing after all. But just knowing what was causing Ryan's behavior and having a name for it bolstered my hopes and gave me the encouragement that I needed to continue on in my efforts to make life bearable for my little son and the rest of our family.

I made a commitment to myself that very day to bury any shreds of pity for myself and for Ryan and to charge full steam ahead in making the best of our situation and learning to cope with and conquer the disability that had been living in our home unidentified for the past nine years.

Chapter 14
He Wouldn't Be that Way If Only . . .

Throughout the past nine years I have struggled with many feelings and emotions. Acknowledging that my little boy was neurologically handicapped was a bitter pill to swallow. Knowing in my heart that it wasn't my fault did not always make the situation any easier to handle. There have been days that I have felt so low that I didn't want to continue on. But love and devotion for my little son has been a much stronger force and always, through all of the trials and tribulations, my love for him and my faith in God have seen me through.

Living with a child with a behavior disorder is hard. Accepting a lifetime of medication for your child is also hard. Knowing that he will never be the policeman or air force jet pilot that he envisions himself is also difficult to accept. The uncertainty of the future is always a concern and trying not to think about it is not always easy.

But through it all, some of the hardest times I have faced have been in dealing with people who have voiced their opinions, sometimes in an offer to help, but many times in a tone of disapproval. Be it stranger or loved one, the criticisms were often directed at Jim and me. In many different ways, however subtle, the message was always the same:

He wouldn't be that way if only. . .

   1. You would spank him more. (Any kid of mine would never act that way and get away with it!)

   2. You would spank him less. (You're too hard on him. Just ignore him and he'll stop!)

   3. You would not allow him to have sugar. (Sugar makes all kids hyper — just cut out the sweets!)

   4. You would not give him red food coloring. (He acts that way because you allow him to have foods with red dye!)

   5. You would give him only fresh foods. (It's the additives and the salicylates that cause hyperactivity!)

   6. You would just give him caffeine. (Haven't you heard that giving black coffee helps hyperactive kids? It's better than all that medication!)

   7. You had sinned less. (It was probably something you did wrong yourself and you're being paid back now by having a child like this!)

   8. You would just pray more. (If you only had enough faith and if you would just pray hard enough, he wouldn't be like this.)

   9. You hadn't let him play with Master's of the Universe toys when he was three years old. (Toys like that are an evil influence.)

   10. You would have the devil cast out of him. (He must be demon possessed!)

   11. You would get a job. (You spend too much time with him.)

   12. You should stay home. (A child like that needs a full-time mother! Quit your job!)

   13. You would give him allergy shots. (Phil

Donohue had a woman doctor on his program that knows exactly how to cure hyperactive kids with allergy shots!)

This list could go on and on. Everyone has an opinion and sometimes those that are the least informed are the quickest to express their thoughts. In the beginning the criticisms would sting, especially before the diagnosis of Tourette syndrome was made. But with adversity I have developed callouses and a gentle ear for those that point their finger. Yet I have learned to be an advocate for Ryan and to intervene when an unthoughtful stranger makes fun of him in public.

On several occasions I have felt compelled to graciously speak to the accusing person, briefly explaining Tourette syndrome and thanking them for their tolerance. I know it will not always be possible to shield him from the many hurts he has yet to face. Even now, a few children at school will taunt him on the playground, laughing at his tics and spreading rumors that he has a disease, some even accusing him of having AIDS. Unfortunately, children at that age do not distinguish one disability from another.

There was one particular day at school that was especially rough for Ryan. He had been having problems keeping his behavior and tics under control that day and a few of the other students, in their childish ignorance, seized the opportunity to tease and make him miserable. Not wanting to let down his "tough guy" exterior, Ryan kept the hurt inside until he got home. Then, like a flooding river, the tears began to flow and the pain he was feeling began to ebb its way out. "Why Mommy, why," he cried. "Why do I have to have this?" "It's not fair," he complained bitterly, with tears pouring down his cheeks. "I HATE this stupid Tourette Syndrome! I just want to be a REGULAR kid. Why can't I just be a REGULAR kid, Mommy?"

As we sat together in the middle of our upstairs hallway, I cradled his limp and sobbing body in my arms. At that moment I would have done anything possible to make his hurt go away. But there was nothing I could do. Yet Ryan, with his heart in tatters, said softly, "Mommy, let's pray right now. Let's ask God to help me be a regular kid." And so we prayed. Ryan, with tear-stained cheeks and the power of a child's faith, prayed that the Tourette syndrome would go away. I too prayed that Ryan would get better, and also that other people would be more understanding and less cruel.

He wouldn't be that way if only. . . how I wish I knew the answer. But if there is one thing of which I am very sure it is of the urgent necessity of a greater public awareness of childhood disorders such as Tourette syndrome and Attention Deficit Disorder. There are hundreds of children and parents suffering these very same hurts and disappointments, but knowledge and support from friends and family would help to make those difficult days a little easier to live!

Being able to share our feelings with members of our families has been a blessing, although there are still a few who refuse to understand. Shedding a tear together with a loved one, or rejoicing over a good day — however big or however small — just knowing that there are others behind us who know what we're going through and who still love us has helped Jim and me through many difficult days.

If only everyone could be more understanding and

patient with children who have behavior problems and their exhausted and rattled parents who are trying to cope! If only. . .

Chapter 15
Angel in Disguise

Love is very patient and kind, never jealous or envious, never boastful or proud, never haughty or selfish or rude. Love does not demand its own way. It is not irritable or touchy. It does not hold grudges when others do it wrong. It is never glad about injustice but rejoices whenever truth wins out. If you love someone, you will be loyal to him no matter what the cost. You will always believe in him, always expect the best of him, and always stand your ground in defending him.
I Corinthians 13:4-7*

The past nine years have been a struggle for all in our family. Having a child with special needs puts a drain on a parent's physical, emotional and spiritual resources. When just getting through the day with a difficult child is a major accomplishment, how then is a parent able to meet the needs of the other "normal" children within the family unit? It's a powerful question with no easy answers.

*Scripture verses are taken from The Living Bible © 1971. Used by permission of Tyndale House Publishers, Inc. Wheaton, Il 60189. All rights reserved.

When my daughter, Julie, was born I had envisioned for her a life with a "Brady Bunch" perfect family. As all parents of a newborn child, I was optimistic that we could offer her a home full of love and a childhood that she could look back on and treasure forever. I never dreamed that the harsh realities of life would deal us such a difficult hand and that she would become an innocent victim of a family in turmoil.

I will always regret that I have not been able to provide Julie with the amount of quality time of sharing that we may have experienced together had circumstances in our lives been different. Ryan's very urgent demands have robbed my daughter and me of the many happy hours that we might have shared together. Many times the strain of having a hyperactive child has sapped my strength rendering me helpless in offering quality time to my other deserving child.

Throughout the past nine years Julie has endured much mental and physical abuse at the hand of her younger brother. Yet somehow she has always managed to have an abundance of love and forgiveness for all the pain he has inflicted. Does she completely understand? I am not sure that she really does, but her love for her family and her brother has resigned her to a life of quiet submission. I wonder, at times, if I would have been the same at her age and I am convinced that I would not. Julie has a very unique quality, a presence in her spirit that allows her to forgive and forget. Despite the abuse and turmoil she has endured, Julie always manages to give Ryan another chance and is very protective of him when others criticize.

We are very proud of our daughter. Julie is an

excellent student and an avid reader. As we watch her enter adolescence we are amused to see new sides emerging in her fun-loving personality and we marvel at her maturity and ability to accept that which she cannot change: her brother's behavior.

Julie, in her twelve short years, has managed to love her brother in the purest form. She has put those verses from the Bible into action without even being aware that she was doing anything special. Yes, to me she is an angel, disguised in the body of a beautiful fun-loving, young girl. As my first-born child, she owns a piece of my heart that can belong only to her. Julie, too, is truly an "exceptional" child.

Chapter 16
One Day at a Time

It has now been seven months since Ryan was diagnosed with Tourette syndrome. I would like to be able to say that our lives have changed dramatically and that Ryan is symptom free; however, learning the correct name for the disability did not magically make everything better. Learning the name of Ryan's disability did, however, give us a sense of peace and has allowed us to come to terms with the prognosis for his future.

Being a child of the "baby boom" generation, I grew up with Dr. Casey and Dr. Kildare working their medical magic on weekly television, and in the back of my mind I always thought there would be a bandaid or a pill that could make everything better. If there is one thing I have learned about Tourette syndrome and Attention Deficit Disorder, it is that there are no easy answers. There is no "quick fix" for these very complicated disorders that plague our children and challenge our parental capacities. But always there is hope for the future and comfort in knowing that there are many ways we can help our children to grow into healthy, happy and independent individuals.

The past seven months have been a sort of roller

coaster with medication changes. Trials of Prozac and clonidine were helpful for a short while; however, in a child's growing body, finding the exact dosages can be a challenge. Ryan is presently taking a combination of Ritalin, clonidine, and haloperidol, some of the most common medications used in the treatment of Tourette syndrome. We have learned to cope with the necessary evil of medications for our little boy, but along with the milligrams of daily medication, comes a megadose of love, hugs, kisses and prayers. We have learned to put up with the swearing and spitting at home in order that he might have the greatest benefit of his medication during school hours when proper social behavior is so critical.

Although Ryan continues to have problems at school, the principal and support staff at his grade school have been wonderful in creating an environment in which he can learn. They have asked for and received information on Tourette syndrome and have put to use the many suggestions from the literature received from the Tourette Syndrome Association. They also speak with Ryan's doctors personally whenever necessary regarding specific problems as they arise.

Jim and I feel very fortunate that Ryan's principal and assistant principal have taken such a positive attitude in working with us and with Ryan's doctors and that they continue to be committed to finding ways for Ryan to progress academically. Ryan continues to be in a regular third-grade classroom and receives approximately one hour of tutoring daily for his difficulties in math, handwriting and reading comprehension. Ryan's principal and teacher allow him to do a large block of his work on a tape recorder, saving him the painful struggle of coping with the difficult task of getting things down on paper. Because of these special interventions and individualized program modifications, Ryan is presently working at grade level in most areas and is progressing nicely.

As you may have guessed, we did change psychiatrists and are presently working with a doctor that has other pediatric Tourette syndrome patients in his practice. The doctor at the City of Hope Medical Center remains our mainstay in prescribing medication and we continue to take Ryan to his regular pediatrician for his routine three month check-ups to monitor his height and weight. Our pediatrician has been very gracious in authorizing referrals for our visits to the doctor at the City of Hope Medical Center after Ryan was finally diagnosed by the two outside specialists, and for that we are very grateful. As for me, I have resolved to never again let a monetary concern on the part of a doctor or health insurance company influence my decision to seek competent and appropriate care for either of my children.

The prognosis for Ryan is good. Inside that little body with the jet engine legs is a spirit of life and a desire to win. His launching crew is in place and all systems are go for a promising future ahead. With a loving family, caring and sensitive physicians, a capable and committed psychiatrist to offer psychological support and a school system that is ready, willing and able to meet the challenges they must face, Ryan has every chance for a bright and happy future.

No, it won't be easy. Until there is a greater awareness of Tourette Syndrome and Attention Deficit Disorder, many children like Ryan will go undiagnosed and untreated. Until there is a better understanding of these disorders these little children and their parents will continue to be criticized and held in low esteem by those from whom they so desperately need love and support.

As I reflect on the past nine years and the struggles we have faced, I am reminded of a poem that I read several years ago that still lies crumpled in my desk. That poem entitled, "Wait and See" was an inspiration to me when I knew in my heart that things were just not right. It compelled me to press on, to not give in, and for the motivation that it sparked in me I am very grateful.

WAIT AND SEE

"There's something here that isn't working.
Does it mean that I am shirking?
Are there answers to my questions?
Who will help my child and me?

"You're too nervous," said her mother,
"Kids are like that," sighed her sister.
"Mine do worse things," moaned her neighbor
And together formed a chorus
"Time will fix it. Wait and See."

To the father she went asking,
"What can we do to help him through?"
"Stop the fussing, Just get to it!
More discipline will get him through it.
He's just like me. Wait and See."

"Neurotic mother," thought the doctor,
"Too concerned for her own good.
This child's healthy, not to worry
Learning's not my cup of tea.
School will fix it, just wait and see."

Off to pre-school, time for playmates
In a group of twentynine
Making friends did not come easy
Cut and paste was work, not fun
The teacher said, "It's maturation.
Wait a year. He'll be just fine."

Kindergarten — learn to listen,
Stand in line and take your turn.
"This child's different. Let's observe him.
Let's not label. . . watch and learn.
Then by next year we will know
If testing is the way to go."

The psychologist was reading
Test results and subtle cues
Of inconsistent learning problems,
Yet to the parents gave the news;
"He isn't far enough behind
To put him in a special class.
We'll offer help the day we find
He's way behind and cannot pass."

Still the story kept unfolding,
Each year losing confidence
Soon the gap was so dramatic

That it had to be addressed
By then the child had mastered failure
The parent had succumbed to guilt.
If only someone had said "Question!
Don't give in! I know there's help!"*

Today, as it did then, the words of that author stir in me a sense of urgency to keep going, to continue to question, and to never give up in finding ways to help my little son. There have been times and instances that I have failed miserably and done and said all the wrong things. I can only trust that my many mistakes have been overcome by my love and devotion.

God has trusted this little life to my care but for a short time. As Ryan continues to grow and my physical influence in his life begins to wane with each passing year, I am becoming ever more aware that there will come a day of independence. As he grows into adolescence many choices will be his, not mine, and I will not always be around to soften the cruel blows that are hurled his way.

As I look toward Ryan's future, I feel at peace knowing that I have given my best to insure his best. I am greatly encouraged in knowing that there are many professionals working to better understand and find new treatments for neurological disorders such as Attention Deficit Disorder and Tourette syndrome.

I hope that Ryan's story has been an inspiration to

*Reprinted from *Their World* magazine with permission of the editor, Julie Gilligan. *Their World* is the annual publication of the National Center for Learning Disabilities, 99 Park Ave., New York, 10016.

you. Today, instead of asking the self-pitying question, "Why me, Lord?" I can sincerely offer a prayer of thanks for the special little child that came into my life. For every heartache, there has been a triumph and as I continue on, taking just one day at a time, I am increasingly grateful for the opportunity and privilege of being Ryan's mother.

Chapter 17
What Is Tourette Syndrome?

Tourette syndrome is an inherited neurological disorder characterized by the presence of tics which usually begin between the ages of 2 to 21. These tics may first appear as unusual movements of the body, such as rapid eyeblinking and head jerking, or as vocal tics such as throat clearing. In some individuals there is compulsive swearing. Other motor tics include, "Hair out of the eyes tics," tugging at clothing, shoulder shrugging, facial grimacing, jumping, touching other people or things, biting oneself, sticking out the tongue, widening of the eyes and mouth opening. Other vocal tics include squeaking, coughing, humming, spitting, grunting, snorting, sniffing, and barking.

In addition to the various tics, there may be other associated behaviors especially Attention Deficit Hyperactivity Disorder (ADHD), obsessive-compulsive behaviors, phobias, learning disabilities, conduct and mood disorders.

Sources of more complete information are given in the Appendix.

Chapter 18
Coping Strategies for Parents

Learning that your child is less than perfect is a tremendous blow to parents. We have all felt compassion for parents of physically handicapped children and empathized with the enormous strain they must face in their day-to-day lives of coping and caring for a handicapped child. Parents of children with Tourette syndrome deserve our compassion and understanding also, but many times instead of sympathy or compassion, they receive criticism and harsh judgements from people who are not aware of the circumstances they face.

Because behavior disorders are many times a part of the complexity of symptoms involved in Tourette syndrome, parents are blamed for their child's inappropriate behaviors by those they encounter in public who are not aware there is a neurological basis for the misconduct. Because children with Tourette syndrome look normal most people assume they are and they are very quick to judge, criticize and blame the poor parents who are often ready to crumble from the daily strain of coping with their child's disability.

Parents of children with Tourette syndrome need to educate themselves about the disorder and absorb as much information as possible in order that they may help to educate those who come in contact with their child. It is not always appropriate to launch into a lengthy dissertation on the latest research on neurological disorders while waiting in the grocery checkout line, but sometimes it helps to politely approach the person who is talking behind your back or shooting poison arrows through the looks in their eyes and to approach them gently with words to the affect: "I am so sorry if my son's behavior has offended you, but he has a neurological disorder called Tourette syndrome and sometimes has difficulty when he's in a busy store or a noisy atmosphere. You can probably imagine how hard it is for all of us, but we're doing the best we can and hope you can understand." Most people when hearing this will change the expressions on their faces faster than Clark Kent changes clothes in the phone booth!

You will find that the majority of people are very understanding, forgiving and sympathetic when approached in a non-confrontive manner. This example accomplishes two things. First and foremost, it gives you an opportunity to discuss Tourette syndrome and create greater public awareness. Many people will respond by saying, "What exactly is Tourette syndrome, I've think I've heard something about it before?" Secondly, it evokes compassion in the other person for not only your child but for you. You can bet that the next time they see a child swearing or knocking over a stool at Burger King they might be more inclined to wonder if the child might have a medical problem instead of thrashing the parental capabilities of the child's parents or condemning the child. It is best if this is done out of ear shot of your child. It's very important that your child not get the idea that you are making excuses for his inappropriate behavior. Being the very perceptive and bright kids that most Tourette children are, this will be a button that they will use to push to keep YOU under their control.

Many parents react to the diagnosis of Tourette syndrome with disbelief, anger, and denial. Others welcome the diagnosis and find great relief that finally there is an explanation for their child's behavior. Some parents will blame themselves or each other, especially when learning that Tourette syndrome can be inherited or passed down from one generation to the next. Some parents refuse to talk about the problem, hoping that it will just go away. Some keep silent from fear of public scrutiny. As parents work their way through these various stages, they will eventually come to the stage of acceptance. It is when they reach this crucial point that they can begin to help themselves and their child.

It is normal to feel resentment at times. Seeing your child's classmates achieving more quickly and realizing that your son will never bring home the "citizen of the month" certificate can be depressing. You may often wonder, why did this have to happen to MY child? What's going to happen when he grows up?

Instead of concentrating on what might have been or borrowing trouble by worrying about the future, it's best to concentrate on the present and to take each day as it comes. No matter how terrible the previous day may have been, start each day fresh with a clean slate for both you and your child. Never mind that YOU may have threatened to run away from home or that he may have become angry and thrown something at you. Each new day should be a new beginning.

A family is like a chain and it is only as strong as its weakest link. Tourette syndrome does not just affect the patient, it affects the whole family and the whole family must learn to adjust to the circumstances on an individual basis. It's important for all family members to keep the lines of communcation open among themselves. Parents should be sensitive to the needs of other children in the family as well as the Tourette child and encourage the siblings to talk about their feelings and frustrations. It's easy for parents to concentrate on the child with Tourette syndrome — they seem to demand more attention than other children, however, spending time individually with each child is very important.

Also, parents need to schedule time away from their Tourette child and take time to be alone as a couple. Burnout is inevitable if parents do not take some time for themselves and allow themselves the luxury of pursuing personal interests or hobbies.

Whenever possible, encourage your child to talk about his frustrations and hurts. He's sure to have them and it's better to help him to get things out in the open instead of festering inside and causing his self-esteem to plummet. Try to make your child's life just as normal as possible. Don't shy away from exposing your child to social situations for fear of public embarrassment. He needs to learn how to cope with his tics and behavior in all situations. After all, he will ALWAYS be your child. The people who glared at you in the department store or restaurant are strangers who you will most likely never see again. Try to always make lemonade out of the lemon situations and make sure that in the end your child's self-worth is still intact.

A child psychologist or child psychiatrist may be very helpful in giving you support through very difficult times. Not only are these professionals able to help your child, but they can also help parents to better cope with seemingly impossible situations. They are trained to help and not to avail yourself and your child of their services during times of need would be unfortunate. Some parents are restricted by health plans or do not have the money needed for this type of help. Most counties have mental health agencies that offer various parenting classes or support groups that may be helpful and sometimes they are provided free of charge or on a sliding-scale fee.

It's a terrible mistake to not be upfront and completely honest with your child's teacher or others with whom he may come in contact, such as the Little League coach or scout leader. Don't be afraid they will label your son or daughter. By not telling them of your child's condition, they may perceive misbehavior to be something it is not: purposeful. Each person that you may help to educate about Tourette syndrome can become an advocate for your child and may help make their road a little easier.

The effects of medication will vary considerably. Check with your child's doctor to learn the possible side effects of any medication they are taking. Some medications will cause your child to tire easily, become more irritable, or to have an increased (or decreased) appetite. Be alert for signs of any new changes in their behavior that may be medication related and report them to the doctor. If your child is on medication, it is wise to keep a diary. If they are going through a trial of various medications or a combination of medications, it is helpful to keep a daily journal or log of the times medications were given and the results noticed. It's much easier and much more accurate when you report back to the doctor at the next phone call or visit. If your child must take medication at school, a watch with multiple alarms may be very helpful. Most teachers will appreciate the child helping to remind them when it's time to go to the office for a pill, and the watch with the alarms pre-set helps your child to feel good about "remembering" their medication.

By becoming informed and educated about Tourette syndrome, parents can begin to help themselves and their child. One way to get information is from your pediatrician; however, new studies regarding symptoms, diagnosis and treatments are emerging quickly and some physicians are not always aware of the newest information regarding Tourette syndrome. Sources of information are listed in the Appendix.

Chapter 19
Ways to Help Your ADHD or Tourette Child at Home

Praise, Praise, Praise! Look for every possible opportunity to give them a word of encouragement. The little things count, too. If they were able to get through the meal without knocking over their glass of milk, make a big deal of it. Always find something to compliment. It will not always be easy but it is so very important to your child's self-esteem to be able to feel your approval.

Don't compare your child with other children. If your child is not achieving at the same level that his brother or sister did, making comparisons only reinforces the child's feelings of inadequacy. Avoid using phrases such as, "Why can't you be like Susie," or "Your brother Michael would never do anything like that."

Encourage them to set their own standards and to work up to their own expectations. Help them to be realistic in their goals. Trying to go two weeks without hitting their sister might be a bit too much. If they should fail on the third day, they will feel like a failure and give up. They may even start hitting their sister even more because in their mind they might reason, "what's the use in trying anyway?" Try taking just a day at a time to begin with.

Try to maintain continuity in their daily schedule. By having mealtimes and bedtimes at the same time each day, you will promote a feeling of security for them and they will feel more comfortable and in control of their environment. Bedtime routines are important and may help your child to fall asleep more quickly. It's best to warn them approximately fifteen minutes before bedtime by saying, "In fifteen minutes it will be time for bed." This gives them time to adjust to the idea of going to bed and does not put you in a confrontive position as you are merely informing them about an upcoming event. Then, about ten minutes later, you might gently say, "Don't forget honey, you have about five more minutes and then I'll help you get ready for bed." This gently reinforces your position and offers your assistance. When the five minutes are up, tell them in a calm but firm voice, "It's eight-thirty now. Time for bed. Would you like to turn off the TV or would you like Mom to do it?" This approach gives them the clear message that they are definitely going to bed, yet it still gives them a choice to make which softens the power struggle between you and them. Hyperactive children should never be in charge of their own bedtimes. If they have difficulty falling asleep, they should still have definite bedtime hours and be encouraged to rest in a quiet atmosphere, even if they cannot always be asleep.

Anticipate! Watch for warning signs of impending anger or blow ups! It may begin with irritability and suddenly escalate into a full-blown explosion! If your child is playing with a game such as Nintendo, for example, and you hear them start to bang the control pad against the chair, or hear frustration in their voice, it's time to step in and suggest that they take a snack break or change to a different game.

Allow them to make their own decisions whenever possible. Children need to feel that their ideas are important and that their feelings count. Try to minimize potential frustrations. Instead of saying, "What would you like for breakfast today?" ask them if they would prefer pancakes or eggs. This limits their choices to only two items and it is much easier and less stressful for them to make a decision.

Don't be afraid to censor their TV time. There are quite clearly television programs that are inappropriate for hyperactive children and ones that tend to fuel their aggressive nature. Even programs as seemingly innocuous as cartoons are sometimes extremely violent and may tend to aggravate these feelings in a hyperactive or Tourette child. It might also be worth considering a boycott of the products that pay for advertising to keep these types of inappropriate shows on the air. One show that is particularly distasteful to me depicts a man with a horribly burned face and a claw for a hand. For children with neurological disorders, some of these types of programs are potentially frightening and disturbing. These children often have a harder time separating fiction from real life and, as Ryan has done, may suffer anxiety and nightmares as a result. We parents need to realize that our purse strings can persuade sponsor's decisions about which programs they will financially support, and we should not be afraid to take an active role in determining what type of shows are allowed to come into our homes for vulnerable little minds to absorb.

Allow them a chance for quiet time. Many children

prefer not to talk much when they come in from school. If they have had a rough day or been the brunt of some unkind teasing, they may not feel like talking about it right away. Always honor their feelings and give them the space they need. Have a "talk" or "sharing" time built into their daily routine if possible. Sometimes this will work best during the dinner hour or at bed or bath time. They may often look forward to that special time and feel much more open and willing to talk about their problems at that time than they would be if you were trying to pry information from them as you're driving home from school.

Fix them nutritious snacks and healthy meals. Avoid junk food and high sugar contents. Encourage them to eat vegetables and fruits instead of cookies and cheese puffs and to drink water, milk or pure juices instead of soft drinks or high sugar fruit punches.

Encourage responsibility in them by providing an opportunity to share in the household chores. Helping you to make a cake can be rewarding for both of you if you resign yourself to not be nervous about the kitchen or the floor. By giving them a chance to measure out the flour and other ingredients, you are creating an opportunity to teach them some very basic math concepts without them even realizing what you're up to! Emptying out the trash baskets, setting the table, and carrying groceries in are just a few of the very basic tasks that they could learn to do with little difficulty. Gradually increase their responsibilities as they are able to handle them, and whenever possible, always allow them a chance to help in deciding which jobs they will do.

Avoid situations that will cause them undue stress

or create a situation for overstimulation. If after a hectic day the family decides that they would like to eat out, for everyone's well-being, please make sure it's a fast food or family restaurant that provides a children's menu and serves their food promptly. It is torture on both of you to drag them into a restaurant with a waiting line only to find that the only entre they offer to children is a quarter-pound piece of rare sirloin on a huge roll with sesame seeds. You're apt to see the lettuce, onion and tomato go flying across the room faster than you can pass the ketchup! As a general rule, keep things simple and it will keep you from losing your mind (and your temper).

Instead of punishment, try finding ways to help your son or daughter gain his or her self-composure. A quiet room, perhaps a "timeout" room will help to separate them from the provoking situation and give them the privacy they need to collect their self control. Be consistent with the time out room after the guidelines have been firmly established. If the child is given five minutes of "timeout," don't talk to them while they are in the time out situation. Set a timer on the kitchen stove and let him know that when they hear the buzzer, they will be able to rejoin the family if they choose to. Remember that five minutes to a hyperactive child can seem like five hours. Keep the timeouts short enough to not seem overwhelming, but long enough to be effective. This takes patience and practice.

Try to say yes whenever possible. If your child asks if they can eat their peanut butter sandwich on the new blue couch, insteading of shouting, "Absolutely not, are you out of your mind?" try to respond calmly by saying, "It would be best if we just eat here at the table. Shall

I get the plates or would you like to?" This accomplishes the same as saying no however, your child is now concentrating on the decision about the plates instead of focusing on the fact that you've actually declined their request to eat on the couch. Whenever possible, offer an alternative when you must reply with a negative answer. Instead of saying, "No you can't go swimming today because it's too cold," you may try something like, "I was hoping you might want to go with me to the video store. You know more about movies than I do. Which do you think would be best, Treasure Island or Old Yeller?"

Show them that your love is abundant and unconditional. It's their misbehavior that you don't like, but you always love them. It's easy to love people who are pleasing us, but it's not easy to show love to someone who is hurting us or acting unkindly toward us. It's never easy to parent a hyperactive or Tourette syndrome child but if you can remember to focus your frustration on this child's behavior and not on the child, it will be much easier to keep those hugs and praises flowing!

Be flexible whenever possible. Try to bend a little whenever possible but don't compromise the rules or your general position. Keeping your child's individual personality in mind will help you to know when it's all right to "fudge" just a little on the rules in a particular situation.

Help them to be independent. Do as much as you can to promote independence in their decision making, but never allowing them the freedom to make decisions that may be dangerous or not age appropriate.

Be firm. If you permeate a feeling of indecisiveness they will pick up on your weakness. Have the fortitude to stand by your convictions and decisions and never let your child bribe or talk you out of something that you know is right for them.

Make sure that the guidelines you have established for them are clear. "Don't throw your socks on the floor," is not the same as saying, "put your socks in the hamper." Say what you mean and mean what you say.

Encourage your family to do things together. If one child is active in sports, try to get all of the children to go to games to offer their support. If your daughter is having a piano recital, her brother should also be there to note her accomplishment and be encouraged to show her his support. Family fun nights such as "Friday Pizza Night" or "Saturday Morning Donut Hikes" can be lots of fun. Even something simple like a family trip to the library or a picnic to a nearby lake or park can be a special time if it is done together.

Praise, discipline, patience, common sense, but most of all, LOVE.

Chapter 20
A Mother Speaks About . . .

BEHAVIOR MODIFICATION — There are many good behavior modification programs that have proven successful with children with ADHD and Tourette syndrome. One thing to be remembered is that no plan is foolproof and no one plan will work all the time. Consistency is the operative word here and no behavior chart or promised reward can elicit model behavior from your child unless you are there to constantly praise and glorify every good deed and each small success.

BOOKS — Until recently available books on Tourette syndrome were virtually non-existent. Good books on Attention Deficit Disorder are hard to find but there are some out there written in language that a lay person can understand. I always check the book stores on each trip to the mall for anything new that may have come in. Some books offer a very biased and slanted view toward various treatment methods. Some are pro medication and some are totally against. I have always found it helpful to read many types of material and then make my own decisions as to its validity. Beware of any books that boast a "cure" or a "quick fix." Some materials written contradict approved medical studies and remain controversial. It sometimes seems that those with the most controversial ideas wind up on the talk show circuit, touting their latest book and leaving a fallout of confusion behind for those of us who have to live with these children on a daily basis.

DADS — Some might think that the father of a hyperactive child is lucky because he gets to escape to work for eight hours a day. Not so. Usually these poor dads get a minute-by-minute replay of everything that happened that day from Mom the minute he walks through the door. Most parents go through the usual stages of denial, anger, guilt and finally acceptance when their child is diagnosed with Attention Deficit Disorder or Tourette syndrome. It's usually the dads who take a little longer to go through each step, sort of like they're in slow motion. Mothers don't get the luxury. They're busy dealing with the pediatrician appointments, making sure the school has pills, having conferences with the teacher and explaining to the principal why her son shouldn't be suspended for tackling the little girl in the pretty pink dress during recess that morning. Fathers can help prevent mothers from burning out by helping out with the "little" things. Jim has been wonderful to help me with the big things like Ryan's homework and getting his bath taken and his clothes on each morning. But sometimes just having him remember to phone in the prescription refills and pick them up is a tremendous help. There have been days when I didn't have the strength or energy to phone Ryan's doctor, and having Jim take over during those times sure helps to reduce the stress.

FAMILY SUPPORT — Support from extended

family or friends is critical in maintaining sanity when dealing with a difficult child. Time away from your child should be scheduled on a regular weekly basis whenever possible and when things are really critical and burnout is burning in your breast; a daily retreat, even for just an hour or so can help. Dealing with a child with a behavior disorder can be overwhelming for even the strongest individual. Trying to cope without support from friends and loved ones is courting disaster. Everyone directly involved with the child should be made fully aware of the problems you are encountering on a daily basis. Providing information to friends and other family members will afford them an opportunity to share in your burden and provide invaluable support to you and your child.

FRIENDS — Friends who understand and accept you and your child, despite the turmoil that you drag along into the relationship, are friends to be treasured for life. So many times people are reluctant to visit or invite you to visit them because of little "you know who." Forget the people who don't understand and try to cultivate and nourish the friendships with those who also don't understand but at least try.

HANDWRITING — Many learning disabled children have difficulty with handwriting or printing and it is especially a concern of children with Tourette syndrome. Many teachers are quick to have a child write sentences or "standards" as a punishment for some misdeed, but for a child with a handwriting disability this is cruel and inhumane punishment! The principal at Ryan's school has been wonderful in helping him with this particular problem. He is now able to do his book reports on a portable tape recorder instead of writing them out. He also answers his test questions verbally instead of struggling to get his answers down on paper. As he becomes more proficient on the computer, it too will offer him an alternative to having to write so much. When some of these small obstacles are removed, we find that many learning disabled children are able to flourish and excel.

IEP MEETINGS — School IEP meetings will be commonplace for parents of children with learning disabilities and for many whose children have Attention Deficit Disorder. The most important thing to remember when receiving notice of an upcoming IEP is to BE PREPARED. If you are unsure of the proceedings, call ahead and ask questions. If you lack confidence in your ability to represent your concerns regarding your son or daughter, ask someone that knows your child well to accompany you to the meeting. Know your rights as a parent and never sign anything that you are not in agreement with. Always take time to study each new recommendation and be sure that you have a clear understanding of what is being proposed. Most IEP meetings are amicable exchanges between parents and school personnel. Should differences occur, keep in mind that nothing is resolved by arguing or bickering. It creates an atmosphere of bad will and is very detrimental to all involved. It's important to remember that you and the school district ultimately have the same common goal — the very best for your child.

MARRIAGE — I do not know how many marriages have crumbled from the undue stress of trying to raise a difficult child. I can only imagine that the numbers are significant. Dealing with the unrelenting emotional upheaval that a hyperactive child can produce can be a strain on even the most solid of marital relationships. If there is not already a solid foundation of love and respect, a hyperactive child may prove to be the wedge that widens the crevice so deep that it can never be repaired. Many parents blame themselves or sometimes each other for the disability in their child. Many are unable to admit that they have produced a child less than perfect and they lash out at the one closest to them — their spouse. Many marriages grow stronger through adversity and Jim and I are fortunate to be in that group. There have been many days when it has been impossible to speak a civil word to each other because of the turmoil of the day, but on those days no words were necessary. We have always remained committed to each other and committed to our son. His pain is our pain and we share it together. For better or worse. Those four little words have taken new meaning since we first spoke them to each other fifteen years ago on a snowy Illinois afternoon.

MEDICATION — If there was ever a subject that should be approached with objectivity, it would be on the issue of the usage of medications in children. As a mother who has seen the best and the worst of both sides of the coin, I can only say that each child is unique and only a competent, qualified physician should make this very critical decision. As children grow, their bodies metabolize medication in a different way and every child who is on medication must be under the very strict guidance of a qualified physician, preferably one who is knowledgeable on the newest diagnostic criteria for childhood neurological disorders. Medications such as

Ritalin remain controversial; however, the benefit/risk factor must be a consideration that parents share with their child's doctor.

MOTHER'S HEALTH — If mom is sick the whole family suffers. We all know that children do not allow mothers to be sick and not even a Super Mom can endure a life of constant physical and emotional abuse from a hyperactive child. It is critical that we moms get enough rest, proper nutrition and a little R&R whenever possible to avoid burnout in the first degree!

PEDIATRICIANS — Having a competent pediatrician or family physician who you can trust is imperative. Not only can the doctor help in diagnosing various neurological disorders, but he aor she may prove a valued source for referrals to any outside professional help that may be necessary. Having a physician who is familiar with your child and family can be a tremendous support and source of comfort.

PETS — To have a pet or not to have a pet? Many hyperactive children, especially those that also have Tourette syndrome, have a tendency to pester or be cruel to pets, even those they care for a great deal. We thought at one time that getting Ryan a dog would be good for him. A child who doesn't have many friends can sometimes benefit from a best buddy: in this case, a small black cocker spaniel named Blackie. Unfortunately, Blackie turned out to be more hyper than Ryan and the two of them together were constant noise and trouble! Although Ryan loved Blackie, his impulsivity prompted him to pester and provoke his little dog and he would often pull his tail, kick him in the side, try to sit on him and throw rocks at him. Blackie was only able to stay with us a few weeks until we decided it would be best to find him a new and safer home. We have since gotten Ryan a small aquarium with four goldfish, which has seemed to satisfy his desire for a pet.

PSYCHOLOGISTS - There are many fine psychologists who specialize in providing therapy for children with Attention Deficit Disorder or hyperactivity. It would also be fair to say that there are also many who are not as knowledgeable in these fields as some of their fellow associates. Long-term therapy for children with these problems is very expensive and, in the opinion of many, unnecessary. I am not at all opposed to psychological therapy. There are many families that definitely need therapeutic intervention and benefit greatly from the help of psychologists. I only urge caution in this area. Once again, your family physician or pediatrician would be best to consult before entering into any long-term or costly therapy sessions.

PSYCHIATRISTS — The services of a child psychiatrist are not necessary in all children with neurological disorders; however, the emotional problems that accompany afflictions such as Attention Deficit Disorder and Tourette syndrome can be devastating to a child and his family. A psychiatrist is a medical doctor who can prescribe medications and sometimes this benefit is to be considered when the necessity for psychological help has been determined.

SCHOOL — Finding an appropriate school program for your child should be of utmost concern. Providing your child with a challenging curriculum in the least restrictive environment while maintaining good self-esteem is essential. Public school systems have many fine programs available for children with special needs, however, accessing your son or daughter to those programs is not always automatic or easy. It's best to contact your local school when you first suspect that your child has a problem. They will refer you to the proper professionals and advise you about the programs available in your local area. It's essential that you familiarize yourself with your state's guidelines for special education as each state has its own individual qualifying criteria.

SELF ESTEEM — Most hyperactive children, or those with learning disabilities, suffer from poor self-esteem. Many cannot cope with their many frustrations and they seem to internalize their failures instead of concentrating on their successes. Many of these children become depressed while others manifest these feelings by becoming angry or lashing out at friends and family. It is a parent's responsibility to ease their child's pain and promote the child's feelings of self-worth by rewarding his or her positive behaviors and showering praise on each success. Even during the most difficult times we must remember to let our child know that it is their misdeed that we do not like, but that we always love them, no matter what may have happened. Hyperactive and learning disabled children need to be reminded of our continuing love for them. Their hearts are like a bottomless pit and we need to keep the love pouring in.

SHOPPING— Don't subject yourself to the humiliation and torture of taking your hyperactive child to the store unless it's an emergency that can't be avoided. Escalators in a mall must beckon with red lights and sirens in the mind of a hyperactive child, for few are able to resist the allure of those shiny moving steps. Until

Ryan was five years old I was able to keep him strapped into a stroller with a wide leather belt, but after that, he was exploring the mannequins, knocking over mirrors, hiding under the racks of clothes and running like FloJo through the fine china department. Occasionally I lose my mind and take him with me, but in my moments of sanity, I take him only when he has to have new jeans or shoes and I need him there to try them on!

SIBLINGS — The brothers and sisters of a hyperactive child have a difficult life indeed. Not only are they often subject to emotional and physical abuse from their hyperactive sibling, they often find it hard to get attention for themselves from their exhausted and sometimes irritable parents! They may bring home a report card of all A's and B's and get a perfunctory, "that's nice honey" from their mom and dad, while little "Johnny Trouble" gets kudos for getting 4 C's and a D! As hard as they try, they just don't always understand why the other kid gets all the attention. It's important to include the other children in the family whenever possible and to let them know exactly what is wrong with their sibling and explain it to them in as much detail as possible. If you don't they may feel angry and resentful. Many times the older siblings take a lot of flak from their friends about their "crazy" or "weird" little brother or sister. They're often embarrassed by their sibling's behavior and concerned that others might perceive the problem to be a sign of mental illness in the whole family. As in most families, sibling rivalry is always a challenge, and sometimes having a hyperactive child in the family complicates this normal childhood occurrence; however, a little of the Cain/Abel syndrome seems inevitable even in the most well-adjusted families.

SNACKS — Anyone with a hyperactive child has probably heard of the Feingold diet and many have tried it. There are still a few die-hards out there that swear it works, but for some strange reason, the medical experts can't seem to prove it and the majority of mothers with hyperactive children can't prove it either! We all know that caffcine perks some people up and others can drink three cups of coffee before bedtime and sleep like a baby. The same analogy can be made with sugar; some children can tolerate it and others can't. I firmly believe that it is important to feed our whole family a healthy diet, including healthy snacks. Eliminating sugar and additives from our child's diet will not eliminate his hyperactivity, but it will help to give him a healthy body. Whenever possible Twinkies and Ding Dongs should be left at the store. Raisins, nuts, sunflower seeds, yogurt, fresh vegetables and fresh fruits are good alternatives to high calorie, high sugar foods that seduce our kids into becoming junk food junkies.

TEACHERS — It helps to remember that teachers are people, too. The majority of teachers are in the classroom today because they love children and they love to teach. It is best to establish a good rapport with your child's teacher at the beginning of the year. Working to keep the lines of communication open is important in helping to assure your child a successful school year. If you feel that your child's teacher is not meeting his or her needs or is insensitive to your child's problems, openly share your concerns. Most teachers are dedicated to the welfare of their students and welcome constructive criticism when presented in a non-threatening manner.

If you and the teacher still seem to be on different wavelengths, perhaps an honest talk with the principal will be productive, however, I feel very strongly that parents should work within the established "chain of command." No teacher appreciates a parent "going behind her back" to the principal, especially about a problem which the teacher never knew existed!

TEMPER TANTRUMS — A hyperactive child has a way of sliding right into the pilot's seat of the family control center, leaving the other family members with a feeling of helplessness. A difficult child will learn from very early on just what buttons to push in dear old mom and dad to get the most reaction. Throwing temper tantrums is usually one way to set off fireworks in a set of parents. Without really meaning to, many parents reinforce the exact behavior they want to extinguish, merely by over reacting and granting the child the attention they are trying to get by displaying inappropriate behavior. It's at times like these that a good behavior modification program will be of great help. Behavior modification programs take the responsibility for misbehavior off the parent and put it directly on the child where it rightfully belongs. Working with your child to encourage and reward good behavior rather than paying attention to or punishing unacceptable behavior is a very workable approach when done in a fair and consistent manner.

TOYS — Hyperactive children need durable toys and games. Quiet toys such as Legos, building blocks, modeling clay and puzzles are all good quiet time activities. Because hyperactive children often have a hard time sitting still for long periods of time, there should also be some action toys available such as a sturdy punching bag or a miniature basketball game. Older children will enjoy tape recorders and walkie talkies and, of course, Nintendo is very popular with all children. I have heard some parents state that Nintendo is very calming for their child, but in our case, I can usually see Ryan's frustration begin to build after ten or fifteen minutes of play and the next thing I know he is throwing the joy sticks at the television screen. Almost all mothers of hyperactive children have to supervise their child's playtime, even if they are left in their room alone. Sometimes it's the quiet moments that are the most dangerous! It's good to be overly cautious with electrical toys, especially if your child has poor impulse control.

VACATIONS — How wonderful it would be to have the perfect family vacation, however, you must not be naive enough to believe that this would ever be possible with a hyperactive child! I remember on one car trip from Cincinnati to Los Angeles Ryan was badgering us with, "how much longer, how much longer" and we hadn't even reached Indianapolis yet. Traveling with children is always a challenge, but traveling with a child like Ryan is a catastrophe. Whenever possible, fly instead of drive. When driving is absolutely necessary be sure to have lots of small travel games handy along with several coloring books and a fresh box of crayons. A cooler full of pint-sized juices and unsalty snack foods are always a good time killer. By the time you get the snacks out and you finish cleaning up what they have spilled all over the car seats, a good half hour has slipped by!

WEEKEND TRIPS— A weekend trip is a great

alternative to a vacation when you have a hyperactive child. We have found that short trips, even one-nighters have been successful in offering the family a chance for some fun. Short trips relieve the stress of many hours on the road and parents stand a good chance at arriving at the motel before their blood pressures reach dangerously high levels! One of the most memorable times we shared as a family was on a short trip to San Diego. It was only a three-hour drive and we arrived early enough that Julie and Ryan could spend a fun day playing in the pool. We had a nice dinner out (a family restaurant, of course) and after dinner took a nice long walk. Before bedtime we all had huge pieces of hot fudge cake, even Mom! We spent the next day at Sea World but came back to the hotel in time for an evening swim before time for bed. After sleeping late the next morning, we had breakfast and headed back to the motel for a quick swim before check out time. We took our time driving home, stopping to look at Old Town and taking a break at the old standby, Mc Donalds. We took another trip much the same to San Francisco the following year and the kids still talk about how much fun we had. We've since had much longer and more expensive vacations but none have been as enjoyable as those two weekend trips.

WORK OR NOT TO WORK—There is a valid argument to both sides of this dilemma. Many mothers feel that it is best for them to stay at home with their hyperactive child on a full-time basis. Other mothers feel that by having an outside interest they are better equipped to withstand the challenges of parenting a hyperactive youngster and that staying home full time would cause them to dwell on their child and his or her difficulties. It was Ryan's pediatrician who first gave me the idea to get a job. I had always felt that I was doing the best thing for him by being home with him every waking minute. But the benefits of a part-time job brought a new freshness to our daily routine. I feel most fortunate to have a job in real estate sales which allows me much flexibility in making my schedule accommodate Ryan's needs. For those mothers who feel overwhelmed by being shut in with a hyperactive child on a full-time basis, a part time job away from your child may be just what the doctor might order!

In this last chapter I have touched just briefly on a few areas common to all mothers of hyperactive children. My suggestions are merely that, suggestions from the heart of a mother who has lived with and loved a hyperactive child for the past nine and one-half years!

Epilogue

Help me Mommy, help me please
There's something in me no one sees
It's hidden in me, hidden well
To look at me, you cannot tell

Others blame you for the things that I do
They think you don't spank me, if they only knew
Our days are not easy, and sometimes you cry
At bedtime we pray, and ask the Lord why?

I hit and I kick you Mom, when I get mad
And after I do it, I feel really sad
I want to stop, but I don't know how
I need to have patience, and I need it NOW!

My friends, they don't always understand
I explain I can't help it, but they think that I can
But I know that YOU love me, both you and Dad
Not only when I'm good, but when I'm bad!

Tourette syndrome, that's the culprit to blame
I don't understand just how it came

It makes me do dumb things called "tics"
I wish it was something the doctor could fix!

I swipe at my hair and I tug at my clothes
And make sure that I kiss you "twice" on the nose
I even things up, and I'm compulsive, you know
Things have to "feel" right to me, be just exactly so

I swear and I scream, and my shriek is so shrill
That you know when it's time for another pill
I'm hyperactive too, I just can't be still
But I'll do better tomorrow Mom,
I PROMISE I will!

I'll make my bed and I'll comb my hair
Brush my teeth? Sure thing, Mom, don't despair
I'll be so good, Mommy, you will see
I promise that tomorrow, I'll be a much better me!

Hit my sister? Nope, NEVER again
We'll play Nintendo together, I'll even let HER win
My teacher; she'll be happy too
When she sees all the things I'm gonna do

I'll pay attention in class, and sit up straight
I'll come in when the bell rings, and not be late
Keep my hands to myself, and be sure not to giggle
I'll be quiet as a mouse, and try hard not to wiggle

I'll be good on the playground, not push, shove or run
I'll take turns at tetherball, and have lots of fun
"Onion" notes? — no more of those for me

A "regular" kid — that's what I'll be

That "regular" kid?, he's inside me somewhere
I can be him some day, with your love and your care
If others would only just give me a chance
Not criticize, judge me, or throw darts with a glance

Not ridicule, laugh, or show faces of scorn
But know I can't help the way I was born!
Just accept it that all of us cannot be
Programmed to act just perfectly

Please help me Mommy, help me to show
Tourettes is an illness, then others will know
That if they would only take time to see
There's a whole lot of wonderful GOOD inside me!

Appendix

Books on Tourette Syndrome:

TOURETTE SYNDROME AND HUMAN BEHAVIOR
by David E. Comings, M.D., City of Hope Medical
Center. 1990, 828 pages, 630 illustrations. Hope Press,
Box 188, Duarte, CA   91009-0188
   For further information about the diagnosis, associated behaviors, cause, genetics, medical and psychological treatment of Tourette syndrome, written for a
general audience, see this companion volume. An order
form is in back leaf.

Organizations:

TOURETTE SYNDROME ASSOCIATION
   42-40 Bell Boulevard
   Bayside, New York 11361
   (718) 224-2999
   This association organizes workshops and sympo-
siums for scientists, clinicians and others working in the
field of Tourette syndrome. It also organizes and assists

local chapters and support groups throughout the U.S. and provides resource information in the form of publications, films and videotapes. Some of the pamplets and videotapes available from the TSA include:

"Coping with Tourette Syndrome — A Parent's Viewpoint," revised, 1981, Elaine Shimberg.

"Coping with Tourette Syndrome in the Classroom," J. Wertheim. revised, 1982.

"Know Your Rights: Facts You Should Know About Your Rights to a Free Appropriate Education." A. Meyers and L. Hammond.

"Tourette Syndrome: The Sudden Intruder" (videotape).

"Matthew and the Tics" (videotape).

"Stop It, I Can't!" (videotape).

LEARNING DISABILITIES ASSOCIATION OF AMERICA (LDAA), previously called ASSOCIATION FOR CHILDREN AND ADULTS WITH LEARNING DISABILITIES (ACLD)

4156 Library Road
Pittsburgh, Pennsylvania 15234
(412) 340-1515

This organization offers membership to parents and professionals and is a national association with both state and local chapters. The national office may provide you with the address of the chapter nearest to your area.

CHILDREN WITH ATTENTION DEFICIT DISORDERS (CH.A.D.D.)
1859 North Pine Island Road
Suite 185
Plantation, Florida 33322
(305) 384-6869 or 792-8100

A non-profit organization that provides information and support to parents who have children with attention deficit disorders. Chapters of Ch.A.D.D. are formed, or being formed, in various locations.

THE ORTON DYSLEXIA ASSOCIATION
724 York Road
Baltimore, Maryland 21204

NATIONAL CENTER FOR HYPERACTIVE CHILDREN
5535 Balboa Blvd. Suite 215
Encino, CA 91316 (818) 986-0514

A non-profit research and treatment center for hyperactive and learning disabled children.

NATIONAL CENTER FOR LEARNING DISABILITIES
This organization publishes a yearly magazine called *Their World.*

Other Books:

THE MISUNDERSTOOD CHILD: A Guide for Parents of Learning Disabled Children, by Larry Silver, 1984,

214 pages. McGraw Hill Book Company, 1221 Avenue of the Americas, New York, New York 10020.

This book explains all facets of learning disabilities, attention deficit disorder and hyperactivity in a very forthright, nonbiased and practical manner. It is written in language that is easy for parents to understand and is very useful and informative. It presents information on the pros and cons of medications and is invaluable reading for parents with children who have any of these disorders.

THE HYPERACTIVE CHILD, ADOLESCENT, AND ADULT: Attention Deficit Disorder through the Lifespan, by Paul Wender, 1987, 162 pages. Oxford University Press, Inc., 200 Madison Avenue, New York, New York 10016.

This book deals more specifically with hyperactivity and Attention Deficit Disorder rather than learning disabilities. Characteristics, causes and treatments are discussed and it is especially interesting to read the chapter on Attention Deficit Disorder in adults.

THE STRONG WILLED CHILD: Birth through Adolescence, by James Dobson, 1978, 240 pages. Tyndale House Publishers, Inc., Wheaton, Illinois 60187.

This excellent book offers practical advice to parents of ADHD children. Quotes in this book were used by permission. All rights reserved.

Index